The Therapeutic Milieu Under Fire

Forensic Focus Series

This series, edited by Gwen Adshead, takes the field of Forensic Psychotherapy as its focal point, offering a forum for the presentation of theoretical and clinical issues. It embraces such influential neighbouring disciplines as language, law, literature, criminology, ethics and philosophy, as well as psychiatry and psychology, its established progenitors. Gwen Adshead is Consultant Forensic Psychotherapist and Lecturer in Forensic Psychotherapy at Broadmoor Hospital.

other books in the series

Forensic Issues in Adolescents with Developmental Disabilities
Edited by Ernest Gralton
ISBN 978 1 84905 144 6
eISBN 978 0 85700 346 1

Therapeutic Relationships with Offenders
An Introduction to the Psychodynamics of Forensic Mental Health Nursing
Edited by Anne Aiyegbusi and Jenifer Clarke-Moore
ISBN 978 1 84310 949 5
eISBN 978 1 84642 890 6

Ethical Issues in Forensic Mental Health Research
Edited by Gwen Adshead and Chris Brown
ISBN 978 1 84310 031 7
eISBN 978 1 84642 396 3

A Practical Guide to Forensic Psychotherapy
Edited by Estela V. Welldon and Cleo Van Velsen
Foreword by Dr Fiona Caldicott, President of the Royal College of Psychiatrists and Helena Kennedy QC
ISBN 978 1 85302 389 7
eISBN 978 1 84642 969 9

of related interest

Mutual Support and Mental Health
A Route to Recovery
Maddy Loat
Community, Culture and Change
ISBN 978 1 84310 530 5
eISBN 978 0 85700 508 3

Professional Boundaries in Social Work and Social Care
A Practical Guide to Understanding, Maintaining and Managing Your Professional Boundaries
Frank Cooper
ISBN 978 1 84905 215 3
eISBN 978 0 85700 446 8

Forensic Focus 34

The Therapeutic Milieu Under Fire

Security and Insecurity in Forensic Mental Health

Edited by John Adlam, Anne Aiyegbusi,
Pam Kleinot, Anna Motz and Christopher Scanlon

Foreword by Kingsley Norton

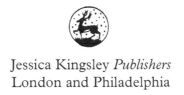

Jessica Kingsley *Publishers*
London and Philadelphia

First published in 2012
by Jessica Kingsley Publishers
116 Pentonville Road
London N1 9JB, UK
and
400 Market Street, Suite 400
Philadelphia, PA 19106, USA

www.jkp.com

Library of Congress Cataloging in Publication Data
The therapeutic milieu under fire : security and insecurity in forensic mental
health / edited by John Adlam ... [et al.] ; foreword by Kingsley Norton.
     p. ; cm.
Includes bibliographical references and index.
ISBN 978-1-84905-258-0 (alk. paper)
I. Adlam, John, 1965-
[DNLM: 1. Forensic Psychiatry--methods. W 740]

614'.15--dc23
                              2011053058

British Library Cataloguing in Publication Data
A CIP catalogue record for this book is available from the British Library

ISBN 978 1 84905 258 0
eISBN 978 0 85700 534 2

Printed and bound in Great Britain

CONTENTS

FOREWORD

Ask a member of the public to imagine a 'secure unit'. She or he may picture neat lines of beds, spotless hospital wards, stately Victorian buildings and rolling acres of land. They might imagine the grounds to be populated by patients busily engaged in productive activities – pathways to recovery and re-entry to society. Those of us who have visited or worked in secure units, however, have our own unique images and memories. I wager that only some of these are characterised by the orderliness, calm and industry of our layperson's imagination.

For many professionals working in secure forensic mental health settings, their environment can be a mystifying and, at times, a frightening place. Frequently it is marked by disorderly and disturbing behaviour, if not outright violence. Staff may not feel adequately supported or supervised and, regardless of profession, they may not feel they have sufficient useful knowledge with which to understand the interpersonal complexities of their workplace (Allen and Jones 2002). At work, ironically, they themselves often feel anything but secure. If you recognise yourself at all in this latter description, this book is a 'must have'. Even if you are not currently working in such an environment but work with patients or clients whose behaviour challenges you (emotionally and/or intellectually), this book is also for you. Should you be my hypothetical member of the public, even you may find something to interest you between the covers of this book. How come such wide appeal?

Well, this book comprises chapters written by a broad range of experts, in a number of forensic and forensic-related fields. All have something pertinent to say about important aspects of forensic clinical practice, much of which is also generalisable to other healthcare settings. Their respective chapters represent distillations of their very considerable clinical experience and expertise. Unusually, some authors provide the reader with insights into their own mental states. Thus you will hear accounts from some who daily find themselves faced with clients or patients, whose dangerous behaviour, abnormal mental states and maladaptive attitudes disturb their own peace of mind, sometimes seriously. You will hear how such professionals (with different background trainings and roles), work under pressures which at times they experience as near intolerable. They describe their struggles to find ways to deal with their clinical (and other professional) encounters. Their aim is to retain (or return to) a respectful and role-appropriate relationship, which avoids emotional detachment from the patient or client and also avoids the perils of over-involvement or inappropriate intimacy – to work in a 'boundaried' manner.

Authors tell of the increased difficulties they experience in fulfilling specific therapeutic roles or applying their particular specialist approach, in the face of uncertainties about the funding and commissioning of their services. They describe the inter-professional tensions and rivalries that surface when money to fund healthcare is scarcer and individual health budgets are, in effect, being reduced. The writers do not shrink from sharing painful details of their striving to maintain morale and to find ethical standpoints from which to view Health Service re-organisation (including that involving unit or service closures) while carrying on working therapeutically. Working under conditions of uncertainty and threat to personal livelihood at the same time as also being exposed to risk of physical violence is, to say the least, uncomfortable. It poses ethical, intellectual and emotional challenges that are painful to experience and hard to process.

Forensic mental health settings are comprised of bricks and mortar but are made up also of myriad interactions and relationships, from the most fleeting to the very long-term, some being measured in decades. In a given day, therefore, countless encounters will take place, many of which could not be claimed to be truly or simply 'therapeutic'. Nonetheless, all actions (or omissions) that involve (or avoid) contact with patients or clients have consequences for those who inhabit these unusual environments. Always, the therapeutic challenge is to structure and organise them, so as to maximise 'good' and minimise 'bad' encounters. Put another way, the aim is to minimise destructive and maladaptive behaviour and attitudes and to promote psychological and social development, which is one definition of the 'Therapeutic Milieu' (Abroms 1969).

To our member of the general public, it might seem strange to specify that an environment embedded within a healthcare setting is 'therapeutic'. Our hypothetical layperson might be forgiven for wondering how any healthcare setting could possibly be anything but! The fact that the term Therapeutic Milieu was coined at all, however, reflects the sad reality that an environment purporting to exist primarily to meet the needs of patients can become overly preoccupied with its own professional issues and performance and, by degree, fail to achieve its primary task of caring (Main 1946). Corrections are therefore required to re-align services and the practices that go on within them, for which various (formal and informal) quality monitoring and inspection processes are needed.

Within the pages of this book, there are plentiful examples of both the intended and unintended effects of recent Health Service changes and re-alignments, some of which have exerted damaging effects on forensic and other highly specialist, forensic-related Therapeutic Milieux. Some of the latter casualties, for example Henderson Hospital, Main House, the Families Unit at the Cassel Hospital and The Arbours Crisis Centre, have been killed off completely, while drastic cuts to psychological therapies are being painfully felt across the forensic field. And, if 'war' is an appropriate metaphor, during this recent period of sustained economic hardship and austerity, we may not yet have seen even the end of the beginning!

Recent changes in government policy, in relation to the organisational changes in the NHS, might be said to have begun years ago, with the adoption of a dominant 'healthcare as business' metaphor and the purchaser/provider split. Some view this as the beginning of a decline in the quality of caring provided within the NHS (Norton *et al.* 1992). To rectify the situation, some are arguing that 'intelligent kindness' within the organisation and delivery of care (which needs to be nurtured at all levels within the system, from policy-makers to clinical staff) is now required (Ballatt and Campling 2011). There is thus an acceptance, in some quarters, that providing professional care now may be more arduous, since professionals no longer enjoy the same degree of trust and respect of former times. There are understandable reasons (relating to professional malpractice and crimes committed against patients) why trust and respect have been eroded. However, some of the loss is due to changes in prevailing societal attitudes and government policies, including the notion that a patient can be simply viewed as a 'customer' – a by-product of professional healthcare being construed as simply another industry.

Providing care and treatment to patients or clients whose pasts are characterised by violent histories (and who themselves were abused or neglected, knowing and inhabiting only insecure attachments), was never and will never be an easy and straightforward business to transact. Such patients and clients often lack the ability accurately to convey their conflicted and contradictory states of mind, which they both house and inhabit. It is as if they firmly believe that their (aggressive, avoidant or seductive) actions will speak to us louder than their words. However, their behavioural expressions of internal states seldom communicate clear and intelligible messages. Consequently, patients continue to feel misunderstood, remaining distrustful, emotionally isolated and insecure. In a complementary position, professionals can feel that they are being kept out of reach and ignorant of their patients' inner worlds. They end up feeling anxious and frustrated (by their patients' defensive behaviour and attitudes), hence de-skilled, demoralised and with little or no sense of therapeutic potency.

As if that were not enough, some of us professionals then give ourselves a good internal beating for not being good enough at our job! This pressure, of internal origin, can impact on our work performance. In the early stages, when pressure is not too high, it may result in our working harder or longer – going that extra mile. However, when that does not deliver – perhaps a smile still does not appear on that patient's face or that line manager's face – the pressure builds still higher. Beyond a certain tipping point, which is different for us all, depending upon both external (interpersonal support networks) and internal (ego/superego) factors, there is a significant (unconsciously defensive) development. That patient or manager who we were (perhaps only unconsciously) trying to please is now our critic, albeit that he or she may not have uttered a single word out of place or have cast an untoward glance in our direction!

What started out, ostensibly, as my personal quest to do well at work, which is a reasonable, even laudable aim, has become 'infected'- something noxious is now in the system. My perception of reality has become profoundly distorted (via the unconscious mechanism of projection, in concert with denial and splitting). What I previously experienced as an internal pressure and injunction to do better and to work harder, I now experience as 'out there' – an unreasonable demand by the external world. Two important aspects are inherent to this dramatic shift in my processing of reality. First, and perhaps surprisingly, I experience some sense of relief. Having a tangible external source of criticism is less hard to handle than an internal 24/7, in-house critic who does not know the meaning of being good enough and does not shut up! Second, I have mistakenly labelled somebody outside as the critic, while the actual (or at least main) culprit is internal – in my mind. This is a significant distortion of reality, which itself potentially evokes further distortions, via the passage of psychic contagion and infection to others in my vicinity.

While some patients, colleagues or managers (on to whom has been projected the punitive aspects of the staff member's superego) do not notice any change in the (projecting) staff member or simply brush off any changes they may have perceived, others do not. Perceiving themselves, for example, to have been distanced, avoided or challenged (unreasonably in their view), they react in a retaliatory and critical manner. This serves to confirm the staff member's original convictions. The scene is thus set for the consolidation of a highly discordant situation. If it is not detected for what it is (the poisonous result of interlocked defensive processes – projective identification), the situation can worsen. Others rally to one or other of the 'wronged' parties, depending on how they evaluate the two sides. What began as an individual staff member's internal problem has very quickly escalated, with the creation of two powerfully opposed and warring sub-systems. In a forensic ward, there are potentially multifarious factions and oppositions: ward staff versus the patients; junior versus senior staff; day versus night staff; one profession versus another; and many more. The most powerfully felt and enduring of opposing factions in forensic settings, for obvious reasons, are those of the staff and patients' sub-systems.

It is because factions usually form along familiar battle lines that they can amass so swiftly. Misleadingly, the speed of formation can also lend credence to the validity of the apparent cause. However, this serves to block a deeper and an enquiring approach to ascertain why this particular battle is being waged at this time or, indeed, at all. Consequently, the ward behaves as if 'content' with this cold (or not so cold) war. Old wounds are re-opened and attempts are made to settle old scores – intra-professional as well as inter-professional. Sadly, the quality of the therapeutic work on the ward is an early casualty. Patients, who may be caught up in the line of fire or indeed may be active participants, may now feel themselves forced into forming closer and more confiding relationships with one another, with which they would ordinarily not have felt comfortable. This can lead to the formation of abusive liaisons, which, because of the prevailing conditions, do not get detected by staff or, if so, do not receive the time and attention required. All of this represents the saving up of future problems for the ward.

The main point to underline here is that the battle can start anywhere in the hierarchy of systems. Even a single internal (ego/punitive superego) spark can ignite the tinder that is the forensic ward – in next to no time, it is all ablaze. However, more heat is generated than light is shed on the original cause. The latter remains unaddressed. Therefore, the potential risk of future fires, from that or any other source, is undiminished. Importantly, an accurate perception of who exactly is 'enemy' and where the firing is coming from is compromised under such circumstances. It is thus as likely that aggressive energy is directed against friend as against foe, which is an extremely worrying situation. This very important topic is amplified in the section of the book devoted to being 'shot by both sides', since a whole organisation can resonate to the warlike themes enacted within one of its sub-systems. Such resonation merely serves to deliver a culture of blame and reinforces divisions.

Helpfully, this book provides examples of destructive processes that originated externally, at the interface between forensic services and the government or others (commissioning and purchasing healthcare services) who are in a position to dictate changes in those services. Regardless of the relevant factors driving the changes, economic and/or ideological, how these changes are implemented, that is, not just what they comprise, is important. The means used to achieve the ends does matter in this field of work. If the implementation of change is carried out without due concern being paid to the people being most affected by it, efficient and successful implementation becomes unlikely. In that event, unintended consequences are more likely to arise, some of which might have been avoided altogether by a more thoughtful introduction of new policy (Norton 2009). As there is usually a stated or, at least, an implied assumption that what is to be changed (by the policy) is fundamentally flawed (ineffective, unfit for purpose or too costly), there is an atmosphere of fault-finding and negativity. In as much as this is unmerited, according to the available evidence, professionals understandably feel the criticism is undeserved, making it much more likely they will not embrace and own the new policy with all its practical implications for them individually.

To avoid such a negative process becoming established and entrenched, managers of services would do well to 'insulate' their clinical workforce from the stated (or implied) criticism associated with policy change, unless in the particular case there is evidence for the failure or fault. In most cases this is not so, therefore managers could recognise the (personal and interpersonal) complexity of the 'change agenda' which is present when clinical staff are being directed to give up and stop working practices and processes that have been part of their professional identity and often cherished by them (Main 1990). Keeping this in mind, managers might provide time and opportunity for discussion and debate, so engaging their workforce more, in an authentic and possibly even a motivated implementation of policy. Such thoughtful management processes would need to be deployed at all levels within a given service undergoing significant change, so as to deliver a genuine embedding of new practices.

The final section of this book outlines some of the potential ways in which individuals, particular services and whole organisations can protect themselves against poisonous and corrosive attacks. It offers a range of potentially helpful frameworks for enquiring into and thereby demystifying the sensitive (interpersonal and inter-systems) world of forensic environments. In doing so, it provides an analysis of the interactions going on between the relevant systems and sub-systems. It suggests what is required in order to propagate healthy survival, within the limits of wider financial support and ideological sympathy. In addition to support from commissioners and rigorous yet sympathetic management style, healthy survival requires the existence of mechanisms. These aim to recognise and deal appropriately with the (often obscured) original sites of critical 'infection', whether deriving from within the healthcare system itself or from without. There is no one-off inoculation to protect professionals against such infective and contagious attacks. However, the instituting of processes such as reflective practice and regular supervision, when implemented with the full support and ownership of the relevant senior (clinical and managerial) personnel, really does contribute significantly to making and keeping the interpersonal environment of the forensic therapeutic milieu a saner and safer place. This is to the benefit of all parties.

Kingsley Norton,
Head of Ealing Psychotherapy,
St Bernard's Hospital, Middlesex

REFERENCES

Abroms, G.M. (1969) 'Defining milieu therapy.' *Archives of General Psychiatry 21,* 553–555.

Allen, C. and Jones, J. (2002) 'Acute wards: problems and solutions.' *Psychiatric Bulletin 26,* 12, 458–459.

Ballatt, J. and Campling, P. (2011) *Intelligent Kindness: Reforming the Culture of Healthcare.* Glasgow: Royal College of Psychiatrists.

Main, T.F. (1946) 'The hospital as a therapeutic institution.' *Bulletin of the Menninger Clinic 10*, 3, 66–70.

Main, T.F. (1990) 'Knowledge, learning and freedom from thought.' *Psychoanalytic Psychotherapy 5*, 1, 59–78.

Norton, K. (2009) 'Understanding failures of NHS policy implementation in relation to borderline personality disorder.' *Psychodynamic Practice 15*, 1, 25–40.

Norton, K., McGauley, G., Wilson, J. and Menzies, D. (1992) 'Health care services in the market place: early effects on caring relationships.' *Therapeutic Communities 13*, 1, 3–26.

ACKNOWLEDGEMENTS

We would like to thank the International Association for Forensic Psychotherapy for providing the frame and the continuity for the series of one-day seminars on which this volume is based. We particularly want to thank Tilman Kluttig, Head of Psychology for Reichenau Hospital in Germany and a past President of the IAFP, for his early encouragement of this project. Several members of the IAFP Board, past and present, have also contributed to this volume. Our special thanks are due to Gwen Adshead, Series Editor for the Forensic Focus Series; Estela Welldon for her tireless work for the IAFP over the last 20 years; and also to Jessica Kingsley for her patience and understanding during the production of this book.

We would like to express our gratitude to the management teams of Broadmoor, Rampton and Henderson Hospitals and the Millfields Unit, John Howard Centre and Respond for jointly hosting this one-day seminar series and to the many practitioners and students who attended and contributed so generously. We hope that they might have learned as much as we did from the experience and from the work collected here. We also acknowledge those many contributors for whose papers we could not find room in this volume.

Lastly, we acknowledge the contribution of the users of services and experts by experience who live in and grapple with their own difficulties in the workplaces described here and especially of those who gave permission for their stories to be recounted at the seminars and in these pages.

EDITORIAL COMMENTARY

This book draws together themes that are central to working with the forensic dilemma in organisational and institutional contexts and settings. It aims to bring to life the thinking of those working on the frontline with highly complex, disturbed, dangerous and endangered people despite the many assaults (conscious and unconscious) that are enacted within the therapeutic relationships and upon the milieu itself.

This volume presents a selection of papers given at a series of one-day seminars, convened between 2005 and 2011, that were jointly hosted by the International Association for Forensic Psychotherapy (IAFP) with Henderson Hospital Services; the Millfields Unit in Medium Secure Forensic Services in East London; two high secure hospitals, Broadmoor and Rampton Hospitals; and Respond, a third sector organisation that works with victims and perpetrators of sexual abuse who live with intellectual disability. The Editors constituted the organising committee for the seminar series over these years. This book marks the end of the first phase of this project and it is also timed to coincide with the 20th anniversary of the founding of the IAFP in 1991.

The aim of the seminar series was to conceive of each event as both a 'stand-alone' inter-professional temporary learning community and as part of an ongoing conversation. The theoretical content of the seminars promoted a psychosocial enquiry into the nature of forensic systems of care and the qualities of their relationship to the excluded outsider. At the end of each day there was a Large Group: a reflective space in which the themes of the event, and their impact, could be processed; in which the relationship between the different memberships of each event could be explored and continuity of purpose within the series could be optimised. If the content of this volume was for the most part generated by the speakers at the various events, this Editorial Commentary and the structure of the book are reflections of the enquiry into the system of care that the large groups made possible.

This seminar series and the discussions within it also occurred at a particular historical moment, a time which saw the closure of numerous well-established and some less well-established centres that used the therapeutic milieu as a central feature in their treatment of people with complex and severe emotional, relationship and behavioural problems. It is fitting that we pause to acknowledge these losses, among them the Henderson Hospital Democratic Therapeutic Community, The Arbours Crisis Centre, Pine Street Day Hospital, The Cassel Hospital Families Service, Main House Therapeutic Community and Webb House Therapeutic Community, to name but a few.

It is beyond the scope of this editorial to comment in detail on the nature of these places, although the contribution of Kingsley Norton's Foreword to this volume, Rebecca Neeld and Tom Clarke's moving clinical account of the work at the Cassel Hospital, and Martin Wrench's personal and professional reflections upon these closures each give a flavour of the extent of these losses and the depth at which they were felt. Andrew Cooper's chapter also examines these themes of loss in his compelling analysis of related political pressure that resulted in the killing off of a therapeutic milieu in a different sort of institution: the profession of social work in the UK.

Although these organisations and institutions do not deliver rapid results, or quick fixes (and do not aim to do so), in ways that can be easily quantified or costed, we consider nonetheless that there is overwhelming practice-based evidence that many people's lives have been transformed by the therapeutic work they have done in such places over the years, as they struggle to make sense of their difficulties and to discover themselves (Turner, Lovell and Brooker 2011). What is equally clear to us is that the lethal attacks that have been carried out against these organisations and institutions all add to a generalised impoverishment of the quality of care for some of our most vulnerable fellow citizens and that it is also a false economy to offer, by contrast, so-called evidence-based, technical-rational packages of treatment under the guise of improving access to psychological therapies.

Indeed, we note with interest that no sooner have we closed these centres of excellence for clinical practice, research and education that the ideas that they promoted begin to rise up again, perhaps more 'acceptably' couched in terms of enhancing 'relational security' (Department of Health 2010) within 'enabling environments', the title of a recent initiative by the Royal College of Psychiatrists. Although we broadly welcome the opportunities that these 'new' initiatives offer, we are concerned that early indications suggest that some of these newly defined spaces are becoming less inter-professional and multi-disciplinary and more 'psychologically informed' in ways that unhelpfully locate professional knowledge within certain types of 'psychological therapists' at the expense of others' more psychosocial understanding or patients' hard-won knowledge and understanding of their own experience.

This volume is conceived in the form of a series of psychosocial and 'groupish' associations (Bion 1961) to the theme of the therapeutic milieu under fire. Our approach is trans-disciplinary and our aim is to invite conversations between service-users, nurses, social therapists, project workers, housing support workers, probation officers, psychiatrists, social workers, group analysts, psychologists, psychotherapists, managers, civil servants, educators, researchers and the general public (among others) about the changing and complex relationship between troubled individuals and their troubling social, organisational and institutional context.

The contributors all work on the 'frontline' in one way or another, many working with marginalised and excluded outsiders at the edges of our exclusive society. This book explores the ways in which these outsiders are offended against and how, in turn, they offend against others, within systems designed both to care for and to contain them. What is the task of the professional caring for a mentally disordered offender? How can they offer security without custody, or care without collusion or detachment? When does 'care' become a perversion of 'control'? Why is thought replaced with action and why might it be so hard for the milieu to replace action with thought? These are some of the central questions that were debated in our one-day seminars, and whose dynamics are explored in this text.

In presenting this range of papers, and the multiple complexities that these authors explore, we hope to enable the reader to come to a better understanding of the ways in which the therapeutic milieu comes under fire from without and within, so that we can think together about how to remain thoughtful and committed to the task while anticipating and responding to these inevitable attacks. Thinking under fire is essential in this work, and so too is reconstructing our internal and external milieux. The systems-psychodynamic thinking of the IAFP and the therapeutic community model combine in contemporary practice to give us a model of the conscious and unconscious processes that inform criminal acting out or the expression of personality disorder: a model that helps us to make sense both of the violence in the patients and the violence in the responses of staff that treat them.

REFERENCES

Bion, W.R. (1961) *Experiences in Groups.* London: Karnac.

Department of Health (2010) *Your Guide to Relational Security: See, Think, Act.* HMSO: Department of Health.

Turner, K., Lovell, K. and Brooker, A. (2011) '"…and they all lived happily ever after": "recovery" or discovery of the self in personality disorder?' *Psychodynamic Practice* *17*, 3, 341–346.

Part I

THE INTERPERSONAL MINEFIELD

THE PSYCHO-SOCIAL DYNAMICS
OF ENGAGEMENT

Infernal world, and thou profoundest Hell
Receive thy new Possessor: One who brings
A mind not to be chang'd by Place or Time.
The mind is its own place, and in it self
Can make a Heav'n of Hell, a Hell of Heav'n.
What matter where, if I be still the same…

Better to reign in Hell, than serve in Heav'n.

From *Paradise Lost*, John Milton (1667)

Chapter 1

NURSING AT THE SCENE OF THE CRIME[1]

Rebecca Neeld and Tom Clarke

In this chapter Rebecca Neeld and Tom Clarke discuss experiences of what they describe as nursing 'at the scene of the crime' at the Families Unit at the Cassel Hospital, now sadly closed down. They describe how traumatised parents managed the difficulties of caring for their children, in what seemed to them like a harsh environment, and the inherent tensions for nursing staff in balancing the therapeutic needs of parents and the health and welfare of their children. They examine the interpersonal minefield between Claire, a young mother of twins, her family and the therapeutic milieu. They focus on the relationship between this family and Margaret, their nurse, to show how the setting of the therapeutic community enabled these dynamics to be thought about (and not thought about) by Claire and Margaret as they grappled with the difficulties they each faced. Neeld and Clarke movingly describe both Margaret's struggle to relate to Claire's experience of being mistreated in her early life (and the ways in which she risked mistreating her own 'at risk' children) and Margaret and Claire's struggle to reach out to the victim and the perpetrator within each of them.

INTRODUCTION

If you were to withhold food, apply restraints so that a person was confined in a chair, left in soiled wet underwear and shouted at repeatedly, you could, if caught in the act, be charged with 'actual bodily harm'. If the person you did this to is your child, the local authority may apply to have your child taken into their care. If you were to contest this decision, one possible outcome used to be that the court could refer you

---

1   An earlier version of this chapter was first presented to the seminar series at the Henderson Hospital Outreach Service in London in 2006 and was later published in *Therapeutic Communities 30*, 4, 412–423 (2009).

and your child to the Families Unit at the Cassel Hospital for assessment and treatment.

Nurses caring for these mothers accompanied by children in the Families Unit not only had to observe these mothers but also had to intersect these abusive and neglectful behaviours of mothers towards their children and intervene. Nurses in these roles therefore had a vicarious experience of the traumas that impacted upon the child. Nurses, like children, prefer to hold on to what is good with the mother (Blum 1981) which is why in order to maintain hope, and possibly to avoid separation, there are occasions when they may turn a blind eye to abuse (see also Chapter 5 and Chapter 10). It is this re-enactment of the trans-generational transmission of trauma, either of what the mother experienced as a child or of what the mother was attempting to repeat with her own child, that the nurse tries to process and resolve within the nurse-patient relationship, in order that this relationship can develop along a different route. Nursing these mothers and their little victims is forensic nursing at the scene of the crime.

BACKGROUND

The individual, group or institution's 'personality' comes about through a combination of experience and the sense that can be made of that experience. The Families Unit's experience was of coming into being after the Second World War. Tom Main, the then medical director, brought his experience and learning gained at Northfield Military Hospital (Harrison 2000) to inform the development of individual psychotherapy and group work to assist individuals to recover from their severely disabling neurotic symptoms. The treatment regime with its emphasis of developing a culture of enquiry and a therapeutic community was extended and broadened to include the treatment of whole families, and the first family was admitted in 1949. From then until the closure of the Families Unit in 2011 there were always babies and children in the building. In the early years it was more usual for these families to consist of a mother who stayed in the Unit and looked after the child and a father who went out to work. Latterly it was more usual to encounter a single mother with a new baby; a mother who often had an older child, or children, already in care.

Rohner (1986) defines abuse as a specialised form of rejection, expressed as the absence or significant withdrawal of warmth and affection of parents towards their children. Such rejection can take the form of hostility and aggression or indifference and neglect. Many of the mothers who came to the Families Unit were extremely vulnerable and yet they had often escaped the attention of adult mental health services. Many had been abused themselves as children (at previous 'crime scenes'); many had self-harmed or used street drugs. Approximately 50 per cent of the women had also spent a period of their childhoods in the care system but it was only when they become mothers that 'the system' started to take notice.

The majority of families, 90 per cent, were referred by the family courts rather than through mental health routes. The mother was usually single (in 80% of cases) and had agreed to come into treatment because she was contesting the social services application to have her child permanently put into foster care, as well as asking for help to stay with and look after her child. The mother may also have neglected her children; a child may have died in suspicious circumstances; older children may have been harmed or malnourished, taken into care or may already be going through the process of being adopted.

The Cassel's particular brand of therapeutic community features individual psychotherapy as a hallmark of its treatment and, prior to the closure of the Families Unit, families and single adults were housed in separate units that came together for community meetings, meals and activities where the full range of society was represented: from babies to grandparents (Kennedy 1987). This coming together of these different strata of society often diluted the intensity that might otherwise develop between individuals when similar sub-groups of people with similar difficulties are in close proximity. The presence of young children running around at teatime or toddlers climbing onto your knee for a cuddle, holding your hand, taking you to see a dead ant, can infuse one with pleasure as well as representing hope for the future: a hope that it might be possible to break the cycle of abuse and rejection. For the hospital itself, the presence of children also signified financial security and perhaps that we were potent and fecund. There was an obvious tension between this sense of growth and potential and the reality of the suffering that preceded and accompanied the presence of children who were 'at risk' in this particular community (as well as the looming socio-economic and political pressures that were increasingly placing the hospital itself 'at risk').

In the wider therapeutic community, the single adult patients often resented the care that the children got, because they didn't have it when they were children. Similarly, a single adult might see a new mother receiving more nursing time than they were getting themselves and feel neglected. Sometimes they refused to participate in helping the new mother to find her feet in the hospital. In these ways, single mothers, and their children, were often the subject of powerful projections from other patients, and from staff, even before they had a name or a history in the therapeutic community. This was often because the compulsory, or coercive, nature of the admission of these mothers also brought the thought (and a reality) of *child-abusers* in a community where 80 per cent of the single adults had experienced abuse and where the abusive nature of patients was often denied and ignored and victimhood claimed or bestowed (Van Velsen 1997; see also Chapter 10). The presence of these mothers with their children who had been harmed brought into stark relief the unavoidable truth that victim-perpetrator roles are often embodied in the same person (Adshead 1997).

THE NURSE, THE BABY AND THE MOTHER

These mothers, as has already been noted, had also been victims (Corby 1993) and were sometimes little more than children themselves and most had not previously had the opportunity of getting help with their capacity to be mothers. The effect that nursing these families had on the nurses was phenomenal. There was the ordinary awfulness of being assaulted with projections that is part and parcel of working with people who have personality disorders who have been subjected to various degrees of childhood trauma. The women could treat the nurses with such contempt, complaining that they were never available, were useless. Perhaps the contempt they manifested was so intense because the mothers felt trapped by their wish to keep the child, as well as their more secret and shameful thoughts that they did not so desire: they were in conflict with competing wishes to be a mother, to be childless and free and without responsibilities and their own 'child-ish' wishes to be looked after. The nurse reaped the consequence of this internal conflict as they tried to respond to these different needs. In order to get to know these young women the nurses had to hear about the children's homes they had been in, the bullying they were subjected to, the total lack of care that they had experienced in ways that generated a great deal of sympathy and warmth as well as the more harrowing tales of their patients' deprivation, neglect and abuse of their own children. The shared task between nurse and patient was perhaps to hold a sense of hope that this time it might be different.

The getting to know each other – nurse and patient, patient and patient – happened within the context of a therapeutic community where nurses and patients managed together the programme of therapeutic 'opportunities', that is, talking, listening, cleaning, cooking, playing and relaxing. For the nurses this often meant being identified with any number of significant others from the mother's past, for example parent, teacher, social worker, police, prison warder and others who may have previously denied them freedom, or removed their children. The internal working model in relation to authority figures of the mothers who contested the removal of their children was naturally one of suspicion and distrust – not helped by the reality that they were in fact being observed and assessed. The mothers may have been abused as children and felt that 'the authorities' had not helped them, or at least not to the extent that made any difference. Establishing a relationship with a woman who hoped to impress upon you her ability to be a good mother, whilst resenting the fact that she experienced your presence as a reminder that she was not a good mother, was of course very difficult and the nurse was often experienced as a kind of critical jailer (see also Chapter 6).

The behaviour of a woman without her children has very little bearing on how she will be when she is with them. Many women who have some degree of personality disorder are able to manage their lives. They have multiple relationships, fall out with people on a regular basis, self-harm, take drugs, drink too much and have difficulty holding down a job for any length of time. But many of these women do not become involved with mental health services until they have children. The longed-for love of another, focused in the baby, does not compensate for the restrictions a baby places upon the mother's tried and tested coping strategies. The mother who at times of stress goes out seeking attention from a man or seeks solace from alcohol will feel impinged upon by their crying babies.

Even when the Families Unit was seen in a good light and as a source of help by the mother, the admission nonetheless did not feel optional or voluntary. It often felt like it was her only way to hold on to her child, or to assert some power over authority figures: an attempt to transform powerlessness into possession and control (Welldon 1988). The nurse usually greeted a new mother whilst awaiting the arrival of her child or children and was often lulled into thinking that the relationship was off to a good start. This time with the nurse and her patient was vital as it was here that the relational bonds were established that helped pull the mother through the times ahead when she came to feel unable to cope with the demands of treatment and motherhood. The patient hopefully felt sufficiently mothered by her nurse to have some mothering to give her baby.

It was not the aim of nursing these mothers to produce a corrective emotional experience. The aim was to help the mothers recognise what they hadn't had and didn't have, so as to help them bear their own deprivation, as well as to manage their envy of their children getting what they did not. The work of nursing the mothers was about being alongside during the trials and tribulations of coping with the restrictions of motherhood and the subjugation of their own needs to their children's needs. In many ways the nurse became the voice of the baby, and so was experienced as a whining, whinging, complaining child. The nurse, when prioritising the baby's needs, could be experienced as if she was disregarding the mother's needs. The care they gave to the baby was felt as the exposure of both a deprived aspect of the mother's past and of her current inadequacies – like putting salt into a wound that had been opened up by the baby's needs.

The nurse needed the mother to work with her, to work towards the outcome of a mother and child going home together, in order that the nurse could feel some potency and a sense of having been helpful. The baby needed the mother. The mother needed the baby. The baby's needs were age-appropriate whereas the mother, wanting to feel loved, replete, fulfilled through having a baby, had needs that were not age-appropriate and were more akin to those of a deprived child. The baby needed to be cared for, fed and contained. Its world needed to be managed in order that it did not feel overwhelmed. The mother had to try to nurse the baby and the nurse had to try to nurse the couple – despite the inherent reciprocal tensions. The nurse might also share very special moments, for example when the baby first walked or talked, but she would also know that the mother would never have wished for her to be the one to share such moments: so the nurses' experiences were often bittersweet.

The nurse in this instance would come to feel like the 'wrong person', simultaneously wanted and pushed away. The nurse might also perceive the mother's individual therapist or social worker to be the preferred one, leaving the nurse feeling deprived and unwanted whilst also having to remain available. These feelings could be understood by the nurse as an experience of something of the mother's own feelings towards those on whom she was dependent.

THE MOTHER

One such mother was Claire, who was herself taken into care at the age of nine years, along with her brother. Claire had been sexually abused by her stepfather, a crime for which he was imprisoned. Her mother had discovered them together and was subsequently admitted to a psychiatric hospital. Claire and her brother were in care for six months before being reunited with their mother. Claire's relationship with her mother deteriorated from the age of 11 and there were further episodes of being looked after by the local authority. Claire's behaviour alternated between being quiet, shy and bullied to being the ringleader, bullying other children. Throughout the latter part of her childhood the longest period she stayed in the same care setting was one year. Claire did remain in contact with her mother but this was intermittent and unreliable.

At the age of 16 years and while still in foster care, Claire gave birth to a baby boy. The child was taken into care and Claire had regular contact with the child during the following year. Claire maintained that she did not know who the father was and suggested that it could have been a number of men. At the time Claire's foster mother reported that she was unaware of any boyfriend of Claire and was not aware that Claire was sexually active. In fact, the foster mother considered Claire might be lesbian as she would get huge crushes on girls at school. By the age of 17 Claire had been rehoused by social services and was living independently, working on a market stall. Contact with her young son had by now broken down.

At 18 years old Claire became pregnant again, this time with twins. Supported by her mother, Claire contested social services' decision to take the twins, Chloe and Anthony, into care and the court directed social services to provide an assessment at the Cassel. Claire was admitted to the hospital when her twins were three months old. She had seen them daily, under supervision, since their birth. Each family came to the Cassel with an entourage of workers. There would be a solicitor, the barrister, the social worker, the guardian *ad litem*, the foster parent. The nurse became familiar with all these participants. With the exception of the social worker, all were in favour of Claire keeping the twins.

Initially, Claire was admitted to the hospital on her own and appeared to settle in well. She joined the other mothers when they sat in the garden to smoke and did not object to sharing a room with another woman who had a baby of ten months. Her introduction to the community meeting was rather more dramatic. An adult patient had cut herself the previous night and been taken to the accident and emergency department. Claire asked the woman why she had done it. Claire said she had tried it but that it didn't do any good and if people really wanted to kill themselves they should be helped to do so. Claire's approach did not win her many friends amongst the adult and adolescent patients but the sentiments reflected the prevailing attitude on the family unit towards people who self-harmed.

THE NURSE

Claire's nurse was Margaret. Margaret had undertaken specialised training in psychosocial nursing at the age of 43 after her own children had left school and following the break-up of her marriage. Previously, she had worked as a general nurse and had worked nights and weekends to fit in with her family requirements.

Training that is informed by psychodynamic and psychosocial perspectives will inevitably raise questions as to one's own motivation to be a care-giver. The type of psychosocial nursing practised at the Cassel is based on the principle that both the patient and the nurse gain (and suffer) within the relationship but not in a way that focuses all the health in one and all the pathology in the other. The degree to which Claire's problems and personal history were to find valences and psychological hooks in Margaret's psyche was to a large extent unknown in the early stages of their working together. Claire was about the same age as Margaret's own daughter and Margaret was of a similar age to Claire's mother. Margaret had said she would like to be a grandmother but not a surrogate mum.

As the primary nurse, Margaret had undertaken a home visit accompanied by a patient representative to Claire, who was then living with her mother and sleeping in the living room. Claire still had her own flat provided by social services and there was the suspicion that she was sub-letting it. Following this first visit, both Margaret and the patient representative reported liking Claire. If there were any anticipated problems, it was thought that Claire would take on the blame for everything that might or could go wrong and would need a lot of support to persevere because of these persecuting feelings.

SCENES FROM THE NURSING RELATIONSHIP: THE BABY, THE MOTHER, THE NURSE AND THE SUPERVISOR

During the first week of Claire's stay, she confided to Margaret that her mother had taken an overdose when Claire was aged ten years. Mother had left an apparent suicide note that Claire found and in which the mother had expressed her inability to see Claire, knowing that the man she loved had found Claire sexually desirable. Mother's feelings made it impossible for her to give Claire the care she needed.

Claire said she felt angry about this and at the same time felt both blamed and responsible. Margaret thought that Claire's androgynous style was to do with keeping herself asexual and undesirable as was Claire's neglect of her self-care and personal hygiene. These were issues which had to be addressed and Margaret would sensitively get Claire to bathe and change her clothes whilst at the same time worrying that her difficulty in caring for herself did not augur well for looking after her children.

The twins arrived and, with a lot of assistance, Claire managed the first three months' assessment period. She was reported to be working in her individual therapy, to be looking after the twins satisfactorily although not playing much with them. The twins appeared to be doing well, were engaged and meeting their age-appropriate milestones. At this point, social services requested the court agree that Claire be treated in her local area, rather than as a residential patient at the Cassel. Claire expressed the wish to stay and after reviewing the local treatment options the Families Unit at the Cassel was able to make a case for Claire to remain. In court, a series of Cassel staff gave evidence as to how well Claire was doing in her treatment and in trying to manage herself and her family. Claire of course heard all these reports and on her return to the Cassel, Claire left the twins with another mother and went out to get drunk. Margaret was on duty at the time and sent Claire to bed on her return and arranged to oversee the twins being put to bed. The next day the staff had to decide what to do. Claire had not been parted from the twins in 14 weeks. Should they be sent to foster care? Did hearing people fight for her bring up feelings about what she didn't have?

The single adult patient who went on the binge drink with Claire was suspended from treatment for a time to allow time for her to reflect on what she had done, but Claire was not suspended and the twins stayed with her. The differences in the treatment and management of different patients were always an ongoing issue in the community. The nurses explained about needing to bear in mind the children's best interests, only to hear a chorus concerning the young adult who had been suspended – how was it in her best interests to be sent away?

The double buggy in which they spent most of their days lost a wheel and Claire's frustration with this was taken out on Margaret:

> I told you it was going to break. Why doesn't the hospital provide me with one, they charge enough, money-grabbing nag bags, always snooping, telling me how I think, feel, fart. I can't stand the bloody place. I want a new nurse.

Margaret came to see her supervisor. She cried, she swore. She said that she hated Claire sometimes. She wondered aloud how the twins would fare when Claire was on rehabilitation. She said that she hated the job then laughed at this. Her supervisor got Margaret some tea. 'I know it's hard,' she said. Margaret stamped her feet and wiped her face. She was told how competent she was and that if the work didn't get to her she would not be as good. Margaret apologised, her supervisor answered that there was no need to: we've all been upset by our patients. Margaret went on to talk about Claire and the homes she had been in, where she was always the second class citizen and treated with contempt. She mentioned how Claire could be so different and asked her supervisor, 'Have you seen her sweet side?' She talked about the small things that Claire had said to her that had made her feel that she was a real person to Claire. For example, Claire found out that Margaret had a love of poetry and bought her a book of poems from a jumble sale. Margaret also reported how dreadful it was to see the boy twin, who she described as less cute and in some ways more demanding than his sister, thrashing about in a temper and trying to get his mother's attention and how Claire would reproach him rather than regard him positively. Margaret confided that she wanted to take him home with her at such times.

Margaret questioned whether she was any good at her job. Should she be more patient? Was she over-critical? If she was a better nurse, would Claire be a better mum to her children? Her supervisor listened and offered what reassurance she could: she felt like the aunty down the road who says, 'Your Mum is having a bad day; it's not your fault'. Margaret was helped to see the patient more clearly and was less contaminated by her own envious and rivalrous feelings. This work of containing the container (Bion 1959) enabled the nurse to continue to nurse her patients. In effect Margaret got the help, in the parallel process that Claire might have benefited from as a child. The nurse's sufficient sense of containment enabled her to return to the patient in a thoughtful state (see Chapter 14). Twenty minutes later Margaret was back talking to Claire about her earlier outburst and about getting a replacement buggy and encouraging her not to keep the twins in it all the time.

Getting Claire to do chores in the community was difficult and as such she was not popular with the single adults in the hospital and so did not have easy access to baby-sitters. At her review it was recommended that she take up a role in the community in order to build relationships with others. In part it was felt that Claire needed to tackle her antagonistic, rude and bullying nature and allow people to see her also as needing help, not as self-sufficient and rejecting of others. She was asked to do the dairy order for the hospital. Claire was erratic in this task; usually she managed to get it done but sometimes Margaret would guiltily do it for her rather than see others go without milk. On one occasion Claire was asked in a community meeting by a fellow patient why her nurse was doing her chores for her. Claire replied that Margaret, like her mother, was a sucker who put up with people who didn't treat them right. Margaret was furious and hurt by these remarks, said to colleagues that she had put up with more than enough and requested that she no longer work with Claire. Margaret had two weeks' leave coming up and the incident was considered in the context of Margaret leaving Claire and the twins but Margaret remained unconvinced. Claire was later told by the community that she should apologise and make reparation.

Claire wrote Margaret an apologetic letter in which she told her how much she meant to her, how she would never have made it this far without her help and how jealous she was of Margaret's own children and their imagined holiday time together. Claire presented Margaret with a picture of the twins and asked Margaret to accept her apology. Margaret did so but added that she was hurt and that it would take time for them to get over this. Margaret also talked to Claire about how her children would fare if Claire treated them like that. Claire didn't see this as a possibility as they were her children and she loved them and would never be like that with them. This lack of insight and the level of denial was worrying for all the team and especially difficult for Margaret who talked a lot about it in supervision and in the nurses' reflective group meetings. An ongoing concern at those meetings was imagining the venom that was redirected at Margaret being directed at the twins.

She talked about how she had felt unable to defend herself, that she felt beaten up and bullied by Claire and how devastated she felt after these continuing onslaughts. We also discussed why no-one defended Margaret at the time of the verbal attack – were we all scared of Claire?

A short time later there was another attempt to challenge Claire in a community meeting and she got up and walked out. She was brought back by another patient, who informed the community that she had seen Claire behave very roughly with her daughter after she had returned from what was described as a 'hard' therapy session. Claire could not bear to discuss this and walked out again. Later, at lunch, Claire was criticised for not clearing up after her daughter, who by this time was nine months old and would fling her food around. A nurse asked Claire to clean up but Claire swore at her, gave her the finger and spat at her. It was evident that Claire was not managing and a meeting was arranged with Claire, her psychotherapist and Margaret following which the children were put into care for a week. During this time Claire remained at the Cassel, continued her treatment and saw her children daily. She said she was worried about being in hospital, that it was relentless and she didn't know if she could 'hack it', and also that she wanted her children back and knew she had to consider them more and to manage her temper.

Margaret considered this a turning point and began to rally support for Claire in the community. She reminded everyone of how delightful the children were and that this should reflect positively on Claire. When Margaret was reminded by other patients of how angry she was with Claire, just a few days earlier, she acknowledged this but added that she also knew how hard Claire's life had been and how hard she tried: as evidenced by her increased ability to keep herself clean and to look after two children. Margaret added that Claire had been there for nine months without a break and that this in itself was hard enough for anyone. Margaret emerged as Claire's champion. She might criticise Claire but was not going to tolerate anyone else doing so. Claire was able to acknowledge her vulnerability for the first time and the community responded with a collective show of compassion. Claire was asked about her own childhood and she responded. An early indicator of a change in relationships in the community was when fellow patients offered themselves as baby-sitters so she could go for an evening out on her birthday. She was praised for not missing a milk order and for helping others. The twins were praised and admired and considered a credit to her. Claire also cried when she talked for the first time about the son she had when she was 16 and the other patients supported her in her wish to re-establish contact and even helped draw up a rota to accompany her on visits.

CONCLUSION

The nurses often found themselves involved with young mothers trying to stay with their child – often their third or fourth child, their other children already adopted or in long-term fostering. The restrictions these mothers felt that their babies imposed upon them often gave rise to hateful, angry, aggressive impulses that were sadistically inflicted on the infants and it was the nurses' job to be positioned between the mother and the child and therefore to intersect with these sadistic impulses. This was to do nursing at a crime scene.

Supervision and staff support was necessary but not sufficient. Both formal and informal structures were required to cultivate the professional awareness of the pitfalls the nurse needed to negotiate in order to maintain hope in the face of adversity. This required that individual nurses had themselves the capacity, as well as the opportunities, to form a secure attachment to the institution.

In such situations the nurse needed also to be attuned to the babies' needs. It was the babies' little shoes the nurse must empathically step into and whose cries she had to translate for the mothers. In giving voice to the babies' needs the nurse was risking the anger that the mother felt from these demands. Sometimes, these identifications set up situations whereby the nurse turned a blind eye to abuse or neglect of the babies because she could not bear to be in these little shoes. Excuses were made. The nurses, like the abused children, often blamed themselves whilst struggling to hold on to the hope it might stop; that next time mum wouldn't choose drugs, drink or men over the relationship with her children.

A major difference between the children and the nurses in the Families Unit, however, was that the nurses had helpful colleagues down the corridor and meetings to attend at given times. Respite was built in to the nurses' day. The nurses were not left with one parent to whom they must cling despite abuse or neglect. The support the nurse received from her colleagues sustained her and facilitated the preservation of hope. Often the hope was illusory and sometimes clearly against the odds: the nurses were hoping for water in a desert without an oasis. Even when there was clearly a need for a separation of the mother and child, the nurses would cling to the hope that the child would be placed in a good home, that they would be adopted and be okay. At such times a blind eye was turned to the statistics about the outcomes for adopted children.

In the Families Unit at the Cassel the prospect of having to stop treatment, to say to the mother, 'No, your baby is to be removed', was close to unbearable and, on the occasions when it did happen, it left us all with a massive emptiness, a sense of failure that was extremely primitive: 'Why was I unable to get this mother to love me and the baby enough to change?' Now that the Families Unit itself is gone, there is a similar mournful lament and a similar dynamic; and across the institution, the organisation and the wider system of care, similar questions are being asked.

REFERENCES

Adshead, G. (1997) 'The Challenge of the Victim.' In H. van Marle (ed.) *Challenges in Forensic Psychotherapy*. London: Jessica Kingsley Publishers.

Bion, W.R. (1959) 'Attacks on Linking.' *International Journal of Psycho-Analysis 40*, 308–315. Reprinted in W.R. Bion (1984) *Second Thoughts: Selected Papers on Psycho-Analysis*. London: Karnac Books.

Blum, H. (1981) 'The Maternal Ego Ideal and the Regulation of Maternal Qualities.' In S. Greenspan and G. Pollock (eds) *The Course of Life: Psychoanalytic Contributions toward Understanding Personality Development, Adulthood and the Aging Process*, vol. 3. Adelphi, MD: US Department of Health and Human Services, NIMH.

Corby, B. (1993) *Child Abuse: Towards a Knowledge Base*. Buckingham, Philadelphia: Open University Press.

Harrison, T. (2000) *Bion, Rickman, Foulkes and the Northfield Experiments: Advancing on a Different Front*. London: Jessica Kingsley Publishers.

Kennedy, R. (1987) 'Work of the Day: Aspects of Work with Families at the Cassel Hospital.' In R. Kennedy, A. Haymans and L. Tischler (eds) *The Family as Inpatient: Families and Adolescents at the Cassel Hospital*. London: Free Association Books.

Rohner, R. (1986) *The Warmth Dimension: Foundations of Parental Acceptance-Rejection Theory*. Beverly Hills, CA: Sage.

Van Velsen, C. (1997) 'The Victim in the Offender in The Challenge of the Victim.' In H. van Marle (ed.) *Challenges in Forensic Psychotherapy*. London: Jessica Kingsley Publishers.

Welldon, E.V. (1988) *Mother, Madonna, Whore: The Idealization and Denigration of Motherhood*. London: Free Association Books.

Chapter 2

THE DYNAMICS OF DIFFERENCE[1]

Anne Aiyegbusi

In this chapter Anne Aiyegbusi explores the dynamics of difference with particular reference to the psycho-social dynamics of race among forensic staff teams. She asks why forensic services may be prone to the creation of therapeutic milieux characterized by painful interpersonal and inter-group challenges that involve various forms of attacks upon those 'other' staff members who are experienced as problematically 'different'. She is centrally concerned with the ways in which this kind of 'nursing at the scene of the crime' mirrors the experiences of patients within the minefields of those services. She elucidates the ways in which difference is identified as the container for toxic projections, and then how, through projective identification, those perceived as 'other' identify with these attributions, becoming helpless, disenfranchised and alienated.

INTRODUCTION

In this chapter, I argue that forensic mental health services have a long history of struggling to provide safe therapeutic care, especially to those patients who are members of minority groups. A surprising aspect of services for mentally disordered offenders is that, despite good intentions and often admirable efforts, progress is usually remarkably slow and difficult to achieve. Some of the struggles to meet the needs of minority groups within services have been evident in the maltreatment and deaths of patients, reaching the public domain in the form of inquiry reports such as *Big, Black and Dangerous* (SHSA 1993), the chapter entitled 'Women in Ashworth' within the Blom Cooper Inquiry into

---

1   An earlier version of this chapter was first presented to the seminar series at the Henderson Hospital Outreach Service in London in 2006 and was later published as a chapter in A. Aiyegbusi, and J. Clarke-Moore (eds) (2008) *Therapeutic Relationships with Offenders: An Introduction to the Psychodynamics of Forensic Mental Health Nursing.* London: Jessica Kingsley Publishers. We are grateful to Jessica Kingsley for giving us permission to reprint a slightly adapted version here.

abuse of patients at Ashworth special hospital (Department of Health 1992) and the Rocky Bennett Inquiry (Department of Health 2003). An unfortunate consequence of reports such as these and the tragedies that precede them is that, on the surface, the ubiquitous problem of discrimination on the grounds of difference gets identified with a small number of isolated services, events and individuals.

Changes that emerge from public inquiries, similar investigations and reviews inevitably focus on structural and social domains. The implementation of strategies to address the behaviour of employees is seen as central to the achievement of change. Much-needed as such action is there is a danger that thought remains the same, only to become enacted at a later date. The observation of particular themes recurring decade after decade suggests a need to also explore the psychological processes that underpin discrimination within forensic institutions (see Chapter 15).

Several authors have argued that social explanations for discrimination on the basis of difference offer an incomplete analysis. Bird and Clarke (1999), Clarke (1999), Dalal (2002) and Frosh (2005) suggest that a deeper psychodynamic understanding is also required in order to achieve a more complete picture of racism, sexism, homophobia and other 'hate' phenomena. They argue that the social expression of prejudice is underpinned by conscious and unconscious psychological processes that are inherent within the human condition. This chapter will describe the psychodynamic processes that are central to understanding human beings' propensity to discriminate against one another, sometimes in hateful, hurtful ways. Why forensic mental health services may be prone to the creation of environments characterized by painful interpersonal relating that usually involve various forms of attacking difference will be explored in this chapter. Nursing processes and practices that aim to work thoughtfully and effectively with the dynamics of difference will also be described.

THE PARANOID-SCHIZOID POSITION

Klein (1946) introduced the concept of the paranoid-schizoid position, an early psychological defence against anxiety whereby the self becomes deeply split into good and bad parts. Good parts represent the life instinct and bad parts are associated with the death instinct. Difference as represented by good and bad parts of the self cannot be held together within the mind because of overwhelming anxiety. In the paranoid-schizoid position, good parts of the self are usually retained but bad parts of the self, which are felt to be unacceptable, have to be evacuated and so are unconsciously projected onto a suitable object, usually but not necessarily another person. The other person who functions as a receptacle for unwanted projections is then experienced as embodying those unpalatable characteristics. This enables the projector to witness their unwanted qualities from a distance, within another who can then be interacted with disdainfully. An example would be of a young man struggling with his sexuality who makes homophobic comments towards a gay acquaintance, insinuating that same-sex relationships are unnatural.

PROJECTIVE IDENTIFICATION

Klein's theory of the paranoid-schizoid position also described the powerful, primitive defence mechanism of projective identification. In projective identification, the person projects 'into' rather than 'onto' another, applying interpersonal pressure until the other experiences the projections as part of themselves. To return to the example of the young man struggling with his sexuality, projective identification could result in his gay acquaintance feeling that his own sexual feelings were abnormal and seeking psychiatric help to 'reverse' the problem. Bion (1959) has described two kinds of projective identification. The first involves communicating mental states to other people; the second can be violent and raw. This involves forcing out unpalatable, unprocessed parts of the self into another until they become felt by the other. Typically, the other is forced to contain uncomfortable emotional states which can be as extreme as terror, rage and murderousness. Bird and Clarke (1999) emphasize the affective nature of projective identification and suggest that, as an interpersonal process, it provides a model for aggressive relating. As such, it may serve as a useful model for understanding the interpersonal transaction between victim and offender. For example, Gary is convicted of attempted murder and detained in a high security psychiatric hospital. In therapy he describes how, when he looked into the eyes of his victim while holding a knife to her throat, he knew that at last somebody understood what it felt like to be him. The forensic patient in this example had been regularly terrorized as a child and had on numerous occasions felt sure that he would be killed during beatings by his violent stepfather. Overwhelmed by his terror and compelled to re-enact his trauma, the only apparent means available for him to communicate this unprocessed experience was by forcing the affect into another person to feel his terror as their own.

HATRED AND OTHERNESS

As Horwitz (1983) points out, when it is understood that through interpersonal interactions people 'may transfer mental contents from one another and back and forth we appreciate the full complexity of behavior in a group setting' (p.269). Not only do people project unwanted parts of themselves into others, but the other can feel and act in accordance with those projections, experiencing them as part of themselves and this can happen between individuals, and within groups and societies on the basis of which cultures are defined. With regard to racism, Fanon (1952) describes the experience of being black and imprisoned in a world constructed by white men. In this world, racist phantasies are intense and through the mechanism of projective identification are forced into black people whose lived experience now concurs with the content of those projections. Thus, the black people who have been projected into then experience themselves as denigrated beings and behave accordingly. In turn this maintains the racist view held by white people. Thus, a cycle of black failure within a white culture becomes perpetuated (see also Chapter 12).

An important aspect of discrimination and bigotry is that by projecting unpalatable parts of the self into a denigrated other, the phantasy of the self as all good is maintained. Therefore, there is an implicit and often necessarily enduring relationship between the projector and their target. One is needed to maintain the psychic equilibrium of the other, which may explain the powerful resistance that tends to accompany efforts to change discriminatory actions on the one hand and thoughts on the other. Change with regard to the latter is rarely even broached, especially in relation to addressing the unconscious processes that maintain oppression on the basis of difference. One reason for this might be that projection operates both at the level of the racist, for example, and among those who serve to challenge racism. In the latter group, it may be more comfortable to think of the other as delinquent while the self is maintained as all good and innocent of any potential for bigotry. Increasing self-awareness would lead to an appreciation of the ubiquity of projection and the fact that everybody unconsciously disposes unwanted parts of themselves onto others in one form or another, especially when exposed to high levels of stress, anxiety or fear. A development, though, has occurred in recent years with regard to race. That is, the allegation of racism now appears to hurt to a degree that it appears to approximate the hurt caused by racist behaviour. Thus, in forensic environments one group of people may be in fear of 'the race card' in the same way that others fear the racist act.

Frosh (2005) has elaborated upon the relationship between projector and target from the perspective of racism and anti-Semitism and suggests that in order for cultures to maintain their civility those parts of the psyche that live within all of us, and may be regarded as primitive but alien, have to be projected into another group for 'civilized' cultures to be maintained. Frosh (2005) goes so far as to suggest that the unconscious longings and desires that inhabit all people are subjectively experienced as alien. What is projected into externally alien groups gives a clue about what our unconscious longings and desires consist of. Generally speaking these projections may include phantasies about socially undesirable indulgences, such as unrestrained hedonism, incompetence, danger, greed, sloth, unbridled sexuality and irresponsibility. Frosh (2005) questions whether this internal, alien part is actually what governs the minds of people rather than the more sophisticated, rational, evolved or conscious part of the human psyche.

This formulation could also explain the relationship between forensic patients and nurses in that the patients may provide a convenient container for nurses' unconscious phantasies, enabling nurses to function more comfortably in the social world. Because they are identified as a group of people who have actually acted out the phantasies other people have, this population may be particularly appealing to the unconscious in terms of serving as repositories for nurses' alien other. For the same reasons, forensic patients as a group who employ primitive defence mechanisms, such as splitting, projection and projective identification, can often be an emotionally difficult population to work with. For the patients, difference has so often served as a target for attack and annihilation as unwanted, internally alien affect is unconsciously deposited in the other. This pattern of interpersonal relating is present within the forensic organization that is uncontained and unable to think about unconscious processes operating within professional groups. In such cases, professionals replicate the style of interpersonal relating that is central to the forensic patients' psychopathology, including attacking and annihilating difference.

One of the factors making caring for forensic patients so complex is that they are victims as well as perpetrators of violence. Therefore, projections are likely to include emotional material associated with victimhood as well as perpetration. The bullying interpersonal transactions that pervade services, often on the part of nurses and other professionals as well as the patient group, can be understood in terms of sado-masochistic functioning. Because nurses work in close proximity to patients, they are often required to process raw and intense sado-masochistic projections (Temple 1996). When nurses are not able to manage this difficult task, they act out on the material, engaging in bullying and discrimination. As such, some nurses adopt the more sadistic role as bully, racist or homophobe for example, while others are on the receiving end of these painful interpersonal interactions.

Case example

Due to chronic nursing shortages, an NHS trust in the UK made a determined effort to recruit a large number of staff from overseas. The NHS trust was located in a part of the country where the population were mostly white and UK born. The newly recruited overseas nurses were not white. Many of these nurses were allocated to work in the local forensic services where nursing shortages had been of particular concern. Their presence was met with emotionally violent rejection and denigration from the patients. The overt abuse and denigration centred on the nurses' physical appearances; that is, those characteristics that were seen as different from their own. Also, the patients on this unit denigrated the overseas nurses' clinical skills as did many of the local nursing staff. Despite having high levels of training and successful careers elsewhere, this cohort of newly recruited nursing staff became hesitant in their work and were reluctant to engage with the patients. As a result, they were further criticized for not being able to do their jobs and became identified within the organization as a group with inferior skills who needed extra supervision.

DISCUSSION

The above case provides an example of how observable difference, on this occasion racial, provides a convenient repository for group projections based on existing feelings of inferiority and denigration within local nurses and the patients. The disorientation of the overseas nurses, who were required to make a huge adjustment to a new country and culture in addition to fresh working arrangements, provided existing, demoralized nurses with an opportunity to be relieved of the emotional burden of feeling devalued and inferior. The overseas nurses also provided the forensic patients with an easy receptacle to contain their hard-to-manage feelings such as fear, vulnerability, alienation and incompetence in terms of failing to succeed in life. Through the application of interpersonal pressure, the overseas nurses began to experience the projected feelings as their own and acted on them, making mistakes and hesitating to get involved with patients. The organization joined in the painful scenario and responded concretely by providing extra supervision. The supervision was not intended to enable the nurses to understand what was going on from a psychological perspective but simply to produce change on a practical or social level in terms of improved performance. In turn, this managerial intervention compounded the discrimination. This example demonstrates how difference can so easily serve as a template for sado-masochistic relating, especially within forensic services as patients and professionals unconsciously seek out receptacles to contain their disturbing feelings.

A THOUGHTFUL APPROACH TO MANAGING THE DYNAMICS OF DIFFERENCE

An alternative scenario to that described in the previous case example might involve a forensic service with commitment to providing a culture of enquiry (Griffiths and Leach 1998) enabling the local nurses, overseas nurses and patients to understand what was going on within their relationships. Community meetings are forums where patients could be challenged about their projections (see also Chapters 1 and 4). For example, in a similar unit where patients were racially abusing a new group of nurses the patients were asked in their community meeting whether having to rely on a new group of nurses for care made them feel particularly vulnerable. Thinking about their feelings of vulnerability in a safe space resulted in some of the patients talking about how worried they were about the new nurses reading their case notes before getting to know them. This anxiety was acknowledged by the group as a whole when one patient was able to explain how frightened he was feeling about being looked after by people he did not know. This patient described having a number of experiences in his life when he had been 'handed over to strangers'. Each experience of simultaneous separation/

introduction felt like a catastrophe. Nurses and patients were able to think about how it would also be easier for the patients to pull the nurses out of their roles rather than wait to be failed by them. Applying so much pressure onto the nurses was one way for patients to take control of their relationships with care-givers. By corrupting the nature of care provided, the patients would be in familiar territory, therefore assuaging anxiety arising from vulnerability.

The new nurses were able to reassure patients that they would organize a number of introductory one-to-one sessions with their primary patients. This would enable the patients to discuss their histories and current needs. The new nurses agreed to involve the patients in any decisions about care plans and would avoid making any radical changes to existing programmes until both parties agreed that a therapeutic rapport had been established. The nurses also clearly communicated the boundaries between their roles and that of the patients, what their authority was and the limits of what would be tolerated in terms of antisocial expressions of distress.

The overseas nurses were supported in their strategy of care by their colleagues. The new and established nurses were able to work as a team in confronting the patients' feelings and behaviour because they had previously been able to explore their own relationships and associated anxieties safely in regular, externally facilitated staff groups. By acknowledging their anxieties together, the two groups of nurses had established common ground, which enabled them to focus on the primary task of delivering healthcare to patients. By remaining on task as a team, progress could also be made with regard to improving the reputation of the service within the wider organization. Nurses were able to recognize that engagement in perpetual conflict enabled them to avoid anxieties associated with the primary task (Menzies Lyth 1988). In forensic mental health nursing, such anxieties arise from close emotional engagement with patients' distress and destructiveness.

By exploring the unconscious processes underlying uncomfortable affect on the part of nurses and patients, what was going on within the social environment was clarified and therefore possible to work with creatively rather than destructively. However, such a challenging task could not have been achieved without a psychologically oriented management team (Obholzer 1994) who approached the appointment and integration of a large group of overseas nurses carefully and with sensitivity to the impact their appointments would have on the patients, the nurses themselves and their colleagues. As such, the action involved in the appointments alone was not seen as the complete solution to the staffing problems. The effective solution required thought on the part of management and the ability to understand the importance of addressing unconscious organizational processes associated with patients' psychopathology as well as observable social behaviour in order to achieve change (Obholzer 1994). Additionally, by being afforded an opportunity to process their feelings together, overseas and local nurses were able to think about hostilities within both groups. By both parties acknowledging their phantasies and feelings of hostility towards each other, as well as their uncertainties and vulnerabilities, neither group was inclined to adopt the role of victim or perpetrator.

TWO TRIBES

The suggestion that discrimination in forensic services only occurs between people who are of different races is to miss the point. While race does appear to provide a particularly convenient receptacle for certain types of projections, it is by no means the only form of difference to emerge as central to in-house conflicts. Gender, sexuality, profession or grade will serve just as well. These apparently tribal conflicts are typical in forensic services for a number of reasons. Forensic patients sometimes function exclusively in the paranoid-schizoid position with extreme use of splitting and projection which is hard for nursing staff to process through thought rather than action. The most obvious split involves the victim/perpetrator dynamic. It is very difficult to integrate the fact that most forensic patients are both victim and perpetrator. The patients themselves have not been able to hold these parts of themselves together in their minds and so the split easily becomes externalized into the environments of forensic services. Typically, conflict within the nursing group gets organized around hard and soft; that is, the hard matter of security and the soft matter of care. These are corollaries to the hard matter of perpetration and the soft matter of victimization.

Because the victim and perpetrator parts of the patient are inevitably split in the patient's mind and indeed often reflected in the structure and organization of services, it may be unsurprising to find that nursing teams tasked with providing care within secure conditions for mentally disordered offenders also find themselves split. However, more than just splitting occurs. The dynamics of difference operate in these environments where hard, security-oriented nurses project their sensitivity and compassion onto and into 'soft' caring nurses who in turn project their sadism and caution into their 'harder' colleagues. Clarke (1996) undertook a covert participant observation into a secure forensic unit and found a typical split within the nursing team; that is, between 'carers' and 'controllers' (p.38). Clarke as part of his research was able to analyse the relationship between carers and controllers within the forensic unit under study. In keeping with paranoid-schizoid functioning, the controllers in Clarke's study were prone to action rather than thought and were not only hostile towards their thoughtful carer colleagues but were also dismissive of care, undermining the staff support group for example. The caring group of nurses in Clarke's study appeared to find their controlling colleagues disturbing but were nevertheless able to consider their own role in maintaining the split.

Clarke's (1996) research identifies one of the key problems in forensic nursing services, which is that as long as such vast splits exist, there is a likelihood that one 'tribe' will never entertain the perspective of the more thinking other. This raises the issue of whether nurses should develop the self-awareness skills necessary to work as professional carers in challenging, emotionally stressful organizations during their pre-registration training (Bray 1998). What seems clear is that in order to address tribal warfare within professional groups in forensic services, support and supervision must be provided to a degree that enables staff to contain the powerful and distressing emotional phenomena projected into them by the patients (Cox 1996). This phenomenon gets organized around difference, and the more visible the difference the more accessible is the target for setting up sado-masochistic relationships which are usually disguised as expressions of legitimate concern.

CONCLUSION

The psychopathology of forensic patients involves the mobilization of primitive defences against anxiety. Nurses who work in close proximity to the patients risk operating in paranoid-schizoid mode too. Exposed to raw, unprocessed projections organized around the victim/perpetrator split in the first instance, nurses are vulnerable to acting out these dynamics and engaging in sado-masochistic functioning if not provided with opportunities to understand the unconscious processes that support this sort of painful interpersonal relating.

In addition to understanding unconscious processes, nurses require supportive, containing structures where they can think about their relationships, test reality and reflect on their experiences thoughtfully.

Increased self-awareness can be developed by integrating reflective spaces such as supervision, staff support or experiential groups into nurses' day-to-day working practice (see Chapters 13, 14 and 15). Through these, the ubiquity of projection and the tendency to offload unwanted parts of the self onto others when under emotional pressure can be explored and contained. By recognizing that vulnerability and sadism exists within all of us, and can and will be externalized within our relationships from time to time, teams are less likely to organize themselves into victims and perpetrators.

When the unconscious is searching for a receptacle within which to deposit the alien, unwanted part of the self, difference provides an appealing container. This dynamic is inherent within the human condition. However, the more psychologically refined a person is, the less likely one might imagine they are to resort to the kind of primitive organization that supports, for example, racist, sexist or homophobic behaviour. The fact that people who would not consider themselves capable of inflicting pain or humiliation on others can find themselves caught up in intense interpersonal conflict within the workplace is what makes forensic services emotionally difficult to work in. Increased paranoid-schizoid functioning occurs when people are highly anxious or frightened. Nurses working in close proximity to disturbed forensic patients are exposed to milieux that are frequently riddled with anxiety and fear. All people within these environments are prone to paranoid-schizoid functioning, particularly when involved in the management of violent incidents. It is perhaps during the anticipation and aftermath of violence that severe sado-masochistic relating which assumes the form of discriminatory thinking and behaviour is most likely to occur.

An important twist to be observed in the dynamics of difference within forensic services is that victims can also be oppressors because the dynamics underpinning the way people relate is ever-present. Unconsciously, the quest to eradicate discrimination can all too often serve as a vessel for sadism. It is for these reasons that promulgation of a culture of enquiry where relationships between staff and patients can be safely explored within containing structures is critical if forensic services are ever to produce lasting change with regard to the difficult atmospheres that have come to define them. That is, change needs to occur below the surface of organizations as well as on top of it and, as such, safely exploring and containing the dynamics of difference would greatly assist the process.

REFERENCES

Bion, W.R. (1959) 'Attacks on linking.' *International Journal of Psychoanalysis 38*, 266–275.

Bird, J. and Clarke, S. (1999) 'Racism, hatred and discrimination through the lens of projective identification.' *Journal of the Psychoanalysis of Culture and Society 4*, 158–161.

Bray, J. (1998) 'Psychiatric Nursing and the Myth of Altruism.' In P.J. Barker and B. Davidson (eds) *Psychiatric Nursing and Ethical Strife*. London: Arnold.

Clarke, L. (1996) 'Covert participant observation in a secure forensic unit.' *Nursing Times 92*, 48, 37–40.

Clarke, S. (1999) 'Splitting difference: psychoanalysis, hatred and exclusion.' *Journal for the Theory of Social Behaviour 29*, 1, 21–335.

Cox, M. (1996) 'Psychodynamics and the Special Hospital: Road Blocks and Thought Blocks.' In C. Cordess and M. Cox (eds) *Forensic Psychotherapy: Psychodynamics and the Offender Patient*. London: Jessica Kingsley Publishers.

Dalal, F. (2002) *Race, Colour and the Process of Racialization: New Perspectives from Group Analysis and Sociology*. London: Brunner-Routledge.

Department of Health (1992) *Report of the Committee of Inquiry into Complaints about Ashworth Hospital*. London: HMSO.

Department of Health (2003) *The Independent Inquiry into the Death of David Bennett*. Cambridge: Norfolk, Suffolk and Cambridgeshire Strategic Health Authority.

Fanon, F. (1952) *Black Face: White Masks*. London: Pluto.

Frosh, S. (2005) *Hate and the 'Jewish Science': Anti-Semitism, Nazism and Psychoanalysis*. Basingstoke: Palgrave.

Griffiths, P. and Leach, G. (1998) 'Psychosocial nursing: A model learnt from experience.' In E. Barnes, P. Griffiths, J. Ord, and D. Wells (eds) *Face to Face with Distress: The Professional Use of Self in Psychosocial Care*. Oxford: Butterworth-Heinemann.

Horwitz, L. (1983) 'Projective identification in dyads and groups.' *International Journal of Group Psychotherapy 33*, 3, 259–279.

Klein, M. (1946) 'Notes on some Schizoid Mechanisms.' In M. Klein (1975) *Envy and Gratitude and Other Works, 1946–1963*. London: Hogarth Press and Institute of Psycho-Analysis.

Menzies Lyth, I. (1988) *Containing Anxiety in Institutions*. London: Free Association Books.

Obholzer, A. (1994) 'Managing Social Anxieties in Public Sector Organizations.' In A. Obholzer and V.Z. Roberts (eds) *The Unconscious at Work: Individual and Organizational Stress in the Human Services*. London: Routledge.

SHSA (Special Hospitals Services Authority) (1993) *Report of the Committee of Inquiry into the Death in Broadmoor of Orville Blackwood and a Review of the Deaths of Two Other Afro-Caribbean Patients: 'Big, Black and Dangerous'*. London: SHSA.

Temple, N. (1996) 'Transference and Countertransference: General and Forensic Aspects.' In C. Cordess and M. Cox (eds) *Forensic Psychotherapy: Crime, Psychodynamics and the Offender Patient*. London: Jessica Kingsley Publishers.

Chapter 3

LIFE ON THE BORDERS OF THOUGHT

Alan Corbett

In this chapter Alan Corbett's focus is on individual psychotherapy with offenders with learning disability and there are powerful implications in what he writes for work with all other forensic patients. Whereas Neeld and Clarke and Aiyegbusi show us the dynamics of engagement in therapeutic milieux through the lens of group, community and team settings, Corbett uses this individual case example to bring out the psycho-social dynamics both in the 'micro' of the therapeutic relationship and in the 'macro' of the fear and hatred of disability 'at the borders of thought' in the wider psychosocial milieu. The story of his work with his patient, Phillip, is an account of grief and violence that are, at least initially, beyond or before words for either patient or therapist. He vividly illustrates the subjectivity of the border established between 'the intelligent' and 'the unintelligent' in the groups, organisations and communities that we construct and the violence that passes between them.

FIRST ENCOUNTER

I go to collect my patient from the waiting area. He looks terrified, his face white, his hands shaking, like a child about to sit on the dentist's chair, as if he is five rather than 50. His support workers encourage him to go into the consulting room with me. Eventually, after much coaxing, he does. I ask him why he thinks he is here. 'To have a walk,' he replies. His voice is gravelly, his words difficult to make sense of. He has large gaps in his teeth, and spittle drips from his mouth as he talks. When I suggest he may be here for something more important than that, he thinks for a while and then suggests: 'to catch up'. He carries with him a sense of never quite arriving in the room and is preoccupied with what his support workers are doing, opening the door every few minutes to peer down the corridor at them, reporting to me what they are doing. I try to engage him in some basic exchanges to build rapport, but to little avail. He is interested in the colours of the walls of the room (a nondescript grey) and the feel of the wall fabric, but seems to find nothing to interest him in the contents of the room – the pens, paints, paper, dolls, or me. He says, 'How are you?' a number of times, his eyes coming to life sporadically, but then dying. I think to myself: 'We have 12 sessions of this' and experience a sinking feeling. I notice a pungent, unwashed smell coming from him, and wish I could be anywhere but here, trying to engage with someone who seems barely able to think, let alone talk, with any clarity.

MAPPING THE VOID

This account comes from the first session of a forensic assessment, and gives a flavour of some of the challenges involved in working with forensic patients who have intellectual disabilities. As forensic psychotherapists, we are mapping new and uncharted territories. In this chapter I wish to navigate my way through a land that holds not just newness, but deep uncertainty. A border is a line separating two political or geographical areas. Maps are political and social constructs in which borders, such as those created between the East and West of Berlin and the North and South of Ireland, are indicators of a particular political judgement made because of particular historical events. Psychological borders, even if not charted on any map, can be just as powerful, such as the invisible line drawn historically between Catholic and Protestant communities in the Falls Road. Life in locations severed by prejudice, fear and hatred places a heavy weight upon all its occupants, whatever side of the divide they live on (see also Chapter 12). In order to carry this weight we may need to deny any fascination with duality of identity in ourselves by adopting a denigration of those on the other side of the border. They become the others of whom it can be thought: 'If they were only like us, all would be well.'

I wish in this chapter to carry this analogy into the realm of forensic psychotherapy with patients with intellectual disabilities as a way of illustrating the subjectivity of the border we have created between the intelligent and the unintelligent forensic patient. I wish also to examine the ways in which forensic psychotherapy with those with intellectual disabilities requires its practitioners to take an intersubjective perspective in order to make sense of the particular colorations, tones and rhythms of disability psychotherapy, making it a journey that not only provides a map of a new area, but brings about a change in our internal map of who we are as forensic psychotherapists and what colours our relationship with our own intelligence.

In doing so, it is useful to reflect on the emergence of an artificial border between forensic psychotherapy with those with intellectual disabilities, and those without. I have described elsewhere (Corbett 2011) the myriad ways in which the psychotherapy profession has neglected the clinical needs of patients with intellectual disabilities. Artificial divisions have been constructed between an 'us' ('mainstream' psychotherapists, forensic clinicians and non-disabled patients) and a 'them' (disability therapists, forensic clinicians treating those with disabilities, and patients who have a disability). This Berlin-type wall creates an annexation of disability therapy in which those working with the disabled operate in a confined territory, rarely visited by those in the larger, non-disabled region. The unconscious fear of engaging with disability may be one factor that tends to ensure that in the confines of an international forensic conference, when faced with choosing to enter a seminar on, for example, working with murderers, perpetrators of incest, borderline patients or patients with disabilities, the first three seminars can be full to capacity, while those signing up for the last seminar can be counted on the fingers of one hand. We can no longer ascribe this enactment of a form of clinical apartheid to the relative newness of psychotherapy with patients with disabilities. It is a discipline that has, in fact, a long and significant history (Corbett 2011; O'Driscoll 2009b) but, it seems, a history that struggles against a collective clinical amnesia, a primitive urge to expel and forget. It may be helpful to locate this phenomenon in the history of psychological therapies and the clinical world's propensity to split, to assume a position of superiority over other modalities in which adherents of a chosen school of thought too easily claim an intellectual superiority over those from other schools (see also Chapter 15).

HISTORY OF FORENSIC DISABILITY PSYCHOTHERAPY

The psychoanalyst Valerie Sinason pioneered the notion of Disability Therapy (Kahr 2000) and its offshoot Forensic Disability Psychotherapy. Her seminal work *Mental Handicap and the Human Condition* (1992; see also Chapter 11) provided a blueprint for working in this field and inspired a new generation of practitioners (Corbett, Cottis and Morris

1996; Cottis 2009; De Groef and Heinmann 1999; Frankish 2009; Freeman 1994; Galton 2002; Hollins and Sinason 2000; Kahr 2000; Linington 2002; O'Driscoll 2009a; Whitehouse *et al.* 2006). Her work with forensic patients encouraged similar initiatives within Respond, the UK's main provider of forensic psychotherapy to patients with intellectual disabilities, and it is from my time as Psychotherapist and Director of this clinic between 1993 and 2003 that the clinical material within this chapter is drawn.

PREVALENCE OF FORENSIC PATIENTS WITH INTELLECTUAL DISABILITIES

Forensic psychotherapy needs to concern itself with patients with intellectual disabilities because they are disproportionately vulnerable to sexual crime – both as victims and as perpetrators. Sobsey (1994) concludes that the presence of a disability produces a likelihood of experiencing sexual abuse that is four times the non-disabled norm. In the UK there are at least 1400 new cases of sexual abuse each year where the victim has a learning disability (Brown, Stein and Turk 1995). Of these cases, 41 per cent of the perpetrators of sexual crimes themselves have intellectual disabilities (the fact that 12% of perpetrators were paid or voluntary carers may be understood in the context of Chapter 5).

There is much debate as to the prevalence of forensic patients with intellectual disabilities in prisons or other secure placements (Holland, Clare and Mukhopadhyay, Simpson and Hogg 2001). A survey of patients in Ashworth, Broadmoor and Rampton secure hospitals posited 16 per cent of patients had an intellectual disability, with one in five having a dual diagnosis of psychiatric disorder (Taylor *et al.* 1998). This is consistent with data on the prevalence of intellectual disability in secure settings in other Western territories (Hayes 2005), with the most comprehensive research in a UK prison concluding that 10.1 per cent of prisoners have intellectual disabilities, with 33.3 per cent falling in the borderline range between mild disability and normal intelligence (Hayes *et al.* 2007). A prevalence rate of 28 per cent has been identified in the Irish prison system (Murphy *et al.* 2000). Given that just over 1 per cent of the general population in most societies have an intellectual disability (Maulik *et al.* 2011), these figures represent a serious challenge to the current paucity of forensic psychotherapy provision for this patient group. The consequences of this therapeutic milieu being under fire may be seen in the disproportionately high rates of abuse and abusing in the lives of intellectual disabilities. It may be possible to conclude that abuse and abusing thrive in a vacuum of specialist or dedicated resources.

UNLOCKING DOORS

Why then are there so many forensic patients with intellectual disabilities and so few forensic disability therapists? Are we still too dutifully bowing to Freud's dictum that a 'certain measure of intelligence' is needed to become a patient in individual analysis (Freud 1901–1905) and Foulkes' (1964) notion that group analysis could only be used by those whose intelligence was 'not below average – preferably high'? If so, we are ensuring not only that the doors to our consulting rooms are closed to neurotic and hysterical patients with disabilities (Bender 1993; Corbett 2011), but that they are locked and bolted against perverse disabled patients. In effect, we are refusing treatment to those who need it most. This chapter opened with the beginning of an assessment that, on its own, may serve to underscore the fears held by many forensic psychotherapists (and other practitioners) about working with this patient group. I wish now to continue with this patient's story in order to examine the narrative themes that emerged following this difficult beginning and, perhaps, to reduce some of those anxieties evoked by the manner of his introduction. I will call him 'Phillip'. All biographical details have been modified for purposes of confidentiality, with consent gained for the sharing of his story.

Case example

Phillip bought with him a long history of attacking women in his home and in his day centre. The women tended to have intellectual disabilities, although there were some reports of him attacking female members of staff as well. His attacks tended to involve placing his hands on the breasts of the women, squeezing them painfully for some time and then running away. He was usually found some time later curled up in the foetal position in a far-flung corner of the home or the day centre, muttering to himself. In hearing this detail I was reminded of Symington's (1988) development of Pierce Clark's (1932) concept of regression to a foetal memory, in which Symington described a retreat to a foetal position as a way of getting back to the womb, at a point before there was prenatal or birth injury.

Phillip's IQ put him at the low to moderate end of the intellectual disability spectrum. He had the capacity (if not always the inclination) to present quite articulately, seeming to understand questions, and was able to say 'yes' or 'no' to them with what appeared to be understanding. His receptive skills, however, were sorely limited, and his seemingly articulate replies masked a massive void, his mind often reminding me of a deep, dark well into which words would be dropped, falling into the void, sometimes reaching the bottom, sometimes not.

His day centre team formed the motor for the referral, consumed as they were with anxiety about the risk he posed to their service users. The group home in which Phillip lived had little of this anxiety, and reported a much lower level of concern as to the danger he presented. His key worker alluded to some concerns about his 'inappropriate behaviour', but described the self-injurious behaviours (such as head-banging and running out into the road) far more than the impact of his actions upon others. In comparing these two polarised versions of Phillip, evidence could be seen of his internal splitting processes being evacuated into and enacted by his staff teams. Phillip, in common with other forensic patients, struggled with a wildly oscillating view of his world as being either all good or all bad – a more nuanced and integrated view of himself, his life and those around him as being a mixture of the good, the bad and the other was impossible for him to adopt. It was unsurprising that those caring for him quickly absorbed this paranoid-schizoid position (Spillius 1996) and acted it out in their polarised views of him and his behaviours. Given the high proportion of disabled patients being supported by different matrices of staff teams, it is inevitable that forensic assessments examine these two locations of splitting – the internal and the external worlds of the patient (Corbett 1996).

These splitting processes were also evidenced through the demand of Phillip's family (his aged father and adult siblings) to be met with separately from the professionals, such was the level of animosity they felt towards anyone charged with his care. They could not bear to be in the same room as some of his workers, leading to a long history of conflict and fragmentation around his case. In both sets of meetings an important question had to be asked, one that had rarely, if ever, been posed: 'How does Phillip make you feel?' For the family, this question uncapped much latent anxiety, hurt and loss that had been there since his birth. His father spoke of his shock at being given the news that Phillip was, in the parlance of the time, handicapped, and feeling as if he was suddenly a handicapped father. I wondered also about the dynamic between Phillip and his now dead mother. Was the experience of the longed-for child suffused with loss? How possible was it for both parents to balance their joy, disappointment, pride and guilt? Phillip's father reacted to these questions with openness, as if an important therapeutic process was beginning to unfold for him too, putting words to feelings that had lain unnamed for many years.

Phillip's teams differed in their responses to this question. Within the day centre staff there was much hostility towards the question itself. It seemed incomprehensible to them that professionals should be asked to analyse feelings in a work meeting. The home team appeared more ready to engage with the question and to explore the very mixed emotions evoked by working with Phillip. Eventually the day centre team more easily accessed their ambivalence towards Phillip, their love and their hate, their nurturing and their fear. It seemed as though progress had already been made in understanding some of what Phillip projected into his external world; the fragmentation and splitting process he all too quickly evacuated into all those around him. The process of integration was by no means a smooth one, and there were times when one or other of the teams experienced significant problems in functioning. This process has echoes of Hopper's (2003) concepts of Incohesion and Massification, whereby the interface between a group of traumatised workers and the trauma of the work itself serves to prevent cohesion, healthy difference and task-related work (see also Chapters 14 and 15).

In my second session with Phillip, following the extremely challenging first session with which this chapter opened, he initially appeared similarly disengaged, and his team reported there had been enormous problems in getting him up that morning. As he came into the consulting room he touched the walls, commenting again on the ridged feel of the wall fabric. We spent some time going over the reasons for his attendance, with a similarly disengaged sense pervading all our exchanges. I asked him about where he lived, what the rooms were like, what he did in each room. At this point something alive flickered in his eyes, and he began talking about his kitchen, the small cooker he used, and the meals his team helped him make. At the end of the session he told me he would bring in some photographs of his home – something I remembered reading in a social work report that he liked to do.

This marked the beginning of a more reciprocal form of relationship between the two of us, and we spent time over the weeks looking through his various Polaroids of his home, and his journey to see me, his cat, and the various members of his support team. I suggested to him we also look at old photographs of his family, a suggestion he liked, and which saw him sharing far more of his personal history with me. He eventually produced photographs of his mother, who had died when he was ten. The pictures of her were much thumbed, and faded through years of being looked at and handled (bringing to mind the obsessional way he seemed to have to feel the fabric of the room's wallpaper).

I commented on this, imagining the hours he had spent gazing at this woman, about whom I knew very little (Phillip's father had refused to answer any questions about his wife – saying she was long dead and buried, there was no point in raking up the past). I commented on the surprise of seeing pictures of Phillip with her. He looked astonishingly different. Clearly a boy with disabilities, but also a boy with life and energy about him – a different person from this worn out, defeated man sitting before me. In one photograph his mother's arms surrounded him, and the young Phillip beamed out from the picture across the years, safe and secure under her wings. The word that came to mind was 'protection', a word I said aloud, adding how sad it must have felt to lose that sense of protection and safety. Phillip grew tremendously sad at this point, holding the photograph firmly in his hand, gripping it tightly as if trying to bring back to life both the woman and the sense of safety she evoked.

Phillip had an obsession with TV soap operas, and told me of storylines he was particularly gripped by. I noticed they all involved physical attacks of some kind, be they robberies, bullying or sexual assaults. He talked about the 'bad boys' in these programmes, and told me he felt they should be locked up by the police for all the bad things they had done. I said that perhaps it was confusing that *he* had not been locked up for the bad things he had done to women. There was a very authentic glint of rage in his eyes as I said this, softened almost immediately by a smile, and the re-emergence of the false self (Winnicott 1960) I had begun to notice. This false self came into play whenever the threat of real connection between us seemed to become a possibility, with him reassuring me he didn't do bad things, and he was not a 'bad boy'.

After this I attempted to explore the notion of bad things being done, and a story began to emerge of bad things being done to him by bad boys (later confirmed as sexual abuse at the hands of older boys in his special school). I linked this to the loss of his protective mother, and again Phillip grew angry, this time at his mother. I commented on how confusing it can be when the person you love lets you down by not protecting you. I was struck by the difficulty he faced in thinking about her death without being overwhelmed by a numbing cloud which he would defend against either through a very brutal shutting down of himself, or a highly charged, enmeshed entanglement with me. Within the course of a number of weeks he grew adhesively attached to me, to the point where he bombarded me with intrusive questions about my marital status, family, home and hobbies. This culminated in a moment that left me with a dizzying mix of shock, intrusion and bafflement when Phillip suddenly drew from his pocket a Polaroid camera with which to photograph me, adding me to his gallery of attachment figures.

DISCUSSION

The words with which we attempt to articulate the most traumatic phenomena reveal as much about ourselves as what we are trying to convey. Language is an important point to consider when thinking about this group of clients. As Valerie Sinason (1992) writes:

> No human group has been forced to change its name so frequently. The sick and the poor are always with us, in physical presence and in verbal terms, but not the handicapped. What we are looking at is a process of euphemism. Euphemisms, linguistically, are words brought in to replace the verbal bed linen when a particular word feels too raw, too near a disturbing experience. (Sinason 1992, pp.39–40)

Thus, perhaps every decade or so, people with intellectual disabilities find themselves facing another name change (and so, too, do those working with them). Working backwards: from intellectual disability to mental handicap to mental retardation to feeblemindedness all the way back to terms like spastic, imbecile and cretin, all of which were perfectly acceptable, social sanctioned phrases of their time. Sinason makes the point that all these terms stem from stupid, which itself stems from stupefied, meaning 'numb with grief'. What emerged through the course of this assessment were two narratives – one of the enactment of sexual violence towards women, one of the near impossibility of processing primary losses of identity, self and sexuality.

One of the challenges of this work is to not collude with a split or polarised view of our patients in which they personify just one of these narratives of victimhood or aggression, rather than both. Taking my photograph was a helpful demonstration of the unconscious's capacity to draw the narratives together. The incident was a troubling one, redolent in its associations of flashing, of sudden assault, and of taking something from another without their consent. I certainly held the conviction throughout my work with Phillip that the levels of containment surrounding him required tightening rather than lessening while I was seeing him, struck as I was by the problems he had with managing impulsivity, and his propensity to sexualise loss in a terribly aggressive manner. He clearly needed a reviewed level of containment around him, groups of people who could talk to each other about him with care and concern, with less fragmentation and more capacity to manage the splitting that is inevitable in working with this patient group. This could help manage his narrative of sexual violence, but alongside this his other narrative, that of loss, damage, the sense of being the unlonged for baby, needed to be held as well.

It is often the case that in working therapeutically with offenders with intellectual disabilities we can find ourselves unable to think, unable to process thought. There are also times when it seems hard for us to speak with any fluency or flow. Our intelligence is under attack, as is theirs. At these moments we are on the receiving end of projections that were too painful for our patients to keep to themselves, namely how hard it is not to be able to talk in the ways that most people talk, and how painful it is to not be able to think as most of the rest of the world think. At such moments we are allowed a painful but important glimpse into our patients' inner worlds, a notion I have described elsewhere (Corbett 2009) as a Disability Transference that is specific to this patient group and that underpins some of the key differences between this work and forensic psychotherapy with the non-disabled.

The notion of two species of forensic psychotherapy – one with patients with intellectual disabilities and one with patients without – is something of a false dichotomy. It is clear to most that all forensic patients possess a form of internal damage that has been most succinctly described in object relational terms by Glasser's (1979) notion of the core concept. Equally, there is at least by analogy a disability countertransference present in other forensic groups and forensic behaviours – sex offenders, self-harm, eating disorders and faecal smearing – where shame, disgust and disappointment may be seen in team and individual responses. This primal developmental attack on the self as the psychogenesis of perversion highlights the importance of viewing intellectual disability through the same theoretical lens with which we view other precursors of sexually aggressive behaviour.

There is, I suggest, more commonality between mainstream and disability forensic psychotherapy than difference. It is in the *frame* rather than the process that differences are contained. It has to be a solid and flexible frame in which to work, allowing the containment of aggressive splitting processes and the integration of those counter-transferential responses that colour so much clinical work with those with intellectual disabilities – fear, hatred, revulsion, pity and disdain. It is to be hoped that as forensic practitioners we have become more comfortable with the notion of discussing and understanding our frightened and frightening responses to the perverse acts of our patients – whether those acts are against others (such as in the sexual abuse or murder of children) or against the self (in the starvation or self-mutilation of the body). Working with patients with damaged brains may make us frightened that our brains won't work well enough. This is a terrifying thought, particularly in a profession that tends to privilege cognition over affect.

The work is intersubjective. It is about two people coming together to discover something about each other. *How* they get to discover each other reveals one of the key differences in this field of work. The distinction lies in the area of rhythm, pacing and tools of communication, rather than in the area of therapeutic or investigative process. The use of creative media is essential when trying to reach and hear forensic patients for whom words are not the main tool of communication. Perhaps the most important tool as clinicians in the field of intellectual disabilities is our self, and our capacity for thinking about what it may be like to not think. Our role thus becomes not just that of auxiliary ego, but of translator. The work is, by definition, long, slow and gradual, and we have an extra role to be explaining this to the outside world, defined as it often is by unrealistic goals and impossible time scales. So, just like our clients, we need to think very creatively about how and what we communicate, and what the limits of words are.

CONCLUSION

If forensic psychotherapy is a relatively young child of psychoanalysis, forensic psychotherapy with the intellectually disabled is a marginalised, ostracised child. Like all children, thinking about its needs involves much consideration of the impact of the child upon ourselves – how as clinicians we deal with the potentially oppressive and suffocating neediness of the unintelligent forensic patient, how we stimulate thought when thought is an indigestible feed and how we remain psychically alive in the face of a seeming psychic death.

The therapeutic milieu that scaffolds and supports Forensic Disability Therapy tends to inevitably be under fire from internal as much as external forces. Savage funding cuts historically attack the sick more than the well, the old more than the young and the disabled more than the able. The survival of this particular milieu is not simply a social and political act, as vital as that is in a time of global recession. It also involves an individual processing of intrapsychic responses to a deficit that, unless analysed and processed, risks our being caught up in a destructive projective process: one in which the primitive terror that is evoked, of our minds being touched by damage, forces us to expel work with this patient group to the margins of our practice. In mapping the differences and similarities inherent in Disability Forensic Psychotherapy, we are inevitably looking afresh at the whole notion of cognitive and affective agency, and realising, I suggest, that the border of thought is a mappable territory in and of itself, and that, as in Berlin in 1989, seemingly immovable walls can be taken down.

REFERENCES

Bender, M. (1993) 'The unoffered chair: the history of therapeutic disdain towards people with a learning difficulty.' *Clinical Psychology Forum 54,* 7–12.

Brown, H., Stein, J. and Turk, V. (1995) 'The sexual abuse of adults with learning disabilities: Report of a second two year incidence survey.' *Mental Handicap Research 8,* 22.

Corbett, A. (1996) *Trinity of Pain.* London: Respond.

Corbett, A. (2009) 'Words as a Second Language: The Psychotherapeutic Challenge of Severe Disability.' In T. Cottis (ed.) *Intellectual Disability, Trauma and Psychotherapy.* London: Routledge.

Corbett, A. (2011) 'Silk purses and sows' ears: the social and clinical exclusion of people with intellectual disabilities.' *Psychodynamic Practice 17,* 3, 273–289.

Corbett, A., Cottis, T. and Morris, S. (1996) *Witnessing, Nurturing, Protesting: Therapeutic Responses to Sexual Abuse of People with Learning Disabilities.* London: David Fulton.

Cottis, T. (2009) *Intellectual Disability, Trauma and Psychotherapy.* London: Routledge.

De Groef, J. and Heinmann, E. (eds) (1999) *Psychoanalysis and Mental Handicap.* London: Free Association Books.

Foulkes, S.H. (1964) *Therapeutic Group Analysis.* London: George Allen & Unwin.

Frankish, P. (2009) 'History and formation of the Institute of Psychotherapy and Disability.' *Advances in Mental Health and Learning Disabilities 3,* 3.

Freeman, A. (1994) 'Looking through the mirror of disability: transference and countertransference issues with therapists who are disabled.' *Women & Therapy 14,* 12.

Freud, S. (1901–1905) *A Case of Hysteria, Three Essays on Sexuality and Other Works.* London: The Hogarth Press and the Institute of Psychoanalysis.

Galton, G. (2002) 'New horizons in disability psychotherapy: the contributions of Valerie Sinason.' *Free Associations 9,* 582–610.

Glasser, M. (1979) 'Some Aspects of the Role of Aggression in the Perversions.' In I. Rosen (ed.) *Sexual Deviation.* Oxford: Oxford University Press.

Hayes, S. (2005) 'Prison Services and Offenders with Intellectual Disability – The Current State of Knowledge and Future Directions.' *4th International Conference on the Care and Treatment of Offenders with a Learning Disability.* University of Central Lancashire.

Hayes, S., Shackell, P., Mottram, P. and Lancaster, R. (2007) 'The prevalence of intellectual disability in a major UK prison.' *British Journal of Learning Disabilities 35,* 162–167.

Holland, T., Clare, I. and Mukhopadhyay, T. (2002) 'Prevalence of "criminal offending" by men and women with intellectual disability and the characteristics of "offenders": implications for research and service development.' *Journal of Intellectual Disability Research 46,* 6–20.

Hollins, S. and Sinason, V. (2000) 'Psychotherapy, learning disabilities and trauma: new perspectives.' *The British Journal of Psychiatry 176,* 32–36.

Hopper, E. (2003) *Traumatic Experience in the Unconscious Life of Groups: the Fourth Basic Assumption: Incohesion: Aggregation/Massification or (ba) I:A/M.* London: Jessica Kingsley Publishers.

Kahr, B. (2000) 'A new breed of clinicians: disability psychotherapists.' *Psychotherapy Review 2,* 2.

Linington, M. (2002) 'Whose handicap? Psychotherapy with people with learning disabilities.' *British Journal of Psychotherapy 18,* 409–414.

Maulik, P., Mascarenhas, M., Mathers, C., Dua, T. and Saxena, S. (2011) 'Prevalence of intellectual disability: a meta-analysis of population-based studies.' *Research in Developmental Disabilities 32,* 419–436.

Murphy, M., Harrold, M., Carey, S. and Mulrooney, M. (2000) *A survey of the level of learning disability among the prison population in Ireland.* Dublin: Department of Justice, Equality and Law Reform.

O'Driscoll, D. (2009a) 'Psychotherapy and Intellectual Disability. A Historical View.' In T. Cottis (ed.) *Intellectual Disability, Trauma and Psychotherapy.* London: Routledge.

O'Driscoll, D. (2009b) 'A short history of psychodynamic psychotherapy for people with learning disabilities.' *Advances in Mental Health and Learning Disabilities 3,* 6.

Pierce Clark, L. (1932) 'The psychology of idiocy.' *Psychoanalytic Review 20,* 13.

Simpson, M. and Hogg, J. (2001) 'Patterns of offending among people with intellectual disability: a systematic review. Part 1: methodology and prevalence data.' *Journal of Intellectual Disability Research 45,* 13.

Sinason, V. (1992) *Mental Handicap and the Human Condition: New Approaches from the Tavistock.* London: Free Association Books.

Sobsey, D. (1994) *Violence and Abuse in the Lives of People With Disabilities: The End of Silent Acceptance?* Baltimore: Paul H Brookes Pub Co.

Spillius, E. (1996) *Melanie Klein Today: Developments in Theory and Practice.* London: Routledge.

Symington, N. (1988) 'The analysis of a mentally handicapped youth: a psychodynamic approach.' *International Review of Psychoanalysis 15*, 8.

Taylor, P., Leese, M., Williams, D., Butwell, M., Daly, R. and Larkin, E. (1998) 'Mental disorder and violence. A special (high security) hospital study.' *British Journal of Psychiatry 172*, 9.

Whitehouse, R., Tudway, J., Look, R. and Kroese, B. (2006) 'Adapting individual psychotherapy for adults with intellectual disabilities: a comparative review of the cognitive-behavioural and psychodynamic literature.' *Journal of Applied Research in Intellectual Disabilities 19*, 55–65.

Winnicott, D.W. (1960) 'Ego Distortion in Terms of True and False Self.' In *The Maturational Process and the Facilitating Environment: Studies in the Theory of Emotional Development.* New York: International UP Inc.

Chapter 4

COMPLAINTS AS A TOOL
FOR BULLYING[1]

Celia Taylor

*In this chapter Celia Taylor examines the way in which the complaints systems
in forensic settings can be subverted or perverted in the cause of attacks upon
staff and upon the therapeutic milieu itself. It is not only the 'psychopathic'
forensic patient who may make perverse use of these systems and Taylor here
sets out some of the ways in which healthcare systems establish rigid structures,
as if to trap their own staff inside their constricting frame, or visit humiliating
retribution in unconscious collusion with the complainant. The psycho-politics
of engagement become fraught and ridden with peril for all parties to the
encounter. Staff are presumed to be guilty until or unless proven innocent and
this is one aspect of the perverse way in which everyone is pushing everyone else
around within the forensic setting. Like Neeld and Clarke, Taylor is writing in
the context of therapeutic community tradition and she also explores how the
milieu can be held and sustained under these prolonged assaults, so that the
complainants can be helped to see that their quasi-judicial 'prosecutions' are
often repetitions of earlier trauma: experiences of grief converted into expressions
of grievance.*

INTRODUCTION

This chapter will examine the complex nature, meaning and emotional
impact of formal complaints by patients against staff in secure settings,
and how one such unit for individuals with 'Dangerous and Severe
Personality Disorder' (DSPD) endeavours to respond to them. It will

---

1   Service user co-presenters contributed to the original talk, on which this chapter
    is based, which was presented at the One Day Seminar, 'Brutal Cultures: Bullying
    and Scapegoating in Forensic Settings', hosted by the IAFP at Broadmoor
    Hospital in May 2010. All service user and staff details in this chapter have been
    anonymised.

also explore how the distress and anxiety generated by such complaints might best be understood and worked with. There is no doubt that robust systems of scrutiny, including complaints procedures, are essential in forensic services, not least because the patients treated within them have forfeited many rights: all are detained under the Mental Health Act, and some have also been sentenced to serve a term of imprisonment – increasingly on an indefinite basis via the new Indeterminate Public Protection orders (Criminal Justice Act 2003; see also Taylor 2011). They lead far from normal lives, locked up often for years (Shaw, Davies and Morey 2001) without leave in secure facilities, where access both to everyday items and people from the outside world is restricted by a range of rules. In the UK, even the right to vote is currently denied to them, in contravention of European law.

Personality disorder units, moreover, have historically been particularly notorious places for abusive practices to flourish. Thus, for example, the Report of the Committee of Inquiry into Complaints about Ashworth Hospital (Department of Health 1992) identified bullying, intimidation, humiliation and the use of physical assault as routine means by which staff exercised control over the patients. Although a reporting system was in place, it was accepted practice that patients' complaints were not upheld. Following a well-meaning drive to overturn this coercive culture, a further inquiry only seven years later found its obverse to be no more desirable (Department of Health 1999). Under the new, 'improved' regime, a blind eye was being turned to patients' access to pornography, illicit drugs and alcohol, as well as to the fact that catalogue fraud and business scams were being run from the ward telephone. Perhaps most damagingly, paedophiles were allowed child visitors. Staff felt powerless to challenge these 'freedoms', for fear of patients' complaints against them, and that these would routinely be upheld by managers.

This swing of the pendulum from one extreme to the other, over a period of only a few years, has been described by Hinshelwood (2002): institutions and the staff that work in them tend to react to personality-disordered individuals in one of two ways. Either there is a greater and greater focus on their 'badness', resulting in increasing degrees of controlling, punitive and fearful behaviour; or there is a tendency to see them as victims of this negative culture, who require sympathy and indulgence: a 'sentimentalised reversal'. Systems of oversight, including complaints processes, need therefore to be highly sensitive both to the nature of the patients and to their impact on the staff working with them.

THE RIGHT TO COMPLAIN

The entitlement to make formal objections when healthcare institutions fall short of their responsibilities has, in fact, only relatively recently been supported by a legal framework. It was not until 1967 that Sir Edmund Compton was appointed by the then Prime Minister, Harold Wilson, to be the first Parliamentary and Health Service Ombudsman, charged with protecting the rights of individual citizens against central government maladministration. In 1972, when the National Health Service (NHS) was undergoing one of its many reorganisations, government policy first introduced the idea of the 'consumer' patient – the intention being that the service would become 'more responsive to the needs and choices of all its users' (NHS Choices 2008). This, perhaps, was the beginnings of a healthcare system in which the satisfaction of the individual was conflated with his or her wellbeing. It was also given a status that potentially put it in conflict with the greater needs of others, since clinicians' ability to prioritise limited resources was compromised. In the new millennium, national standards were introduced with the publication of an NHS Plan (Department of Health 2000), to be overseen by an independent inspectorate, the Commission for Health Improvement (CHI). This body has now been replaced by the Care Quality Commission (CQC). Arguably, responsibility for shortfalls in the NHS was thus located in the workforce rather than in central government.

Since 2009 all Trusts have been required to operate a formal procedure for investigating complaints, and a year later the right to complain was incorporated into the NHS Constitution (Department of Health 2010). The NHS web site (www.nhs.uk) now lists no fewer than ten different organisations that those who believe themselves to have been badly treated can approach. These include clinicians' professional regulatory bodies, which have the power to remove rights to practice and thus careers and livelihoods (for the other side of this coin, see Chapter 5). Information and advice for patients and their families on how to complain about any aspect of the service with which they are dissatisfied is frequently prominently displayed in hospital foyers and wards. These procedures have even given rise to a new breed of 'complaints professional' (Lester *et al.* 2004) to oversee the process and ensure that it is carried out efficiently.

According to the NHS Constitution for England (2010), the goals of the complaints procedure are to ensure that any complaint is properly investigated and dealt with efficiently, and to inform the complainant of the outcome. If the complainant is still dissatisfied, he or she can appeal to the independent Parliamentary and Health Service Ombudsman. Compensation payments are promised to those who have been 'harmed', although what constitutes harm and who decides whether it has been inflicted is not defined. But, as was vividly illustrated by events at Ashworth Hospital, complaints procedures can be very ineffective at achieving these goals in a way that achieves a balance between protecting both patients and staff, or that results in better care.

A DEFENCE AGAINST BETRAYAL

Very seldom do these procedures formally consider that complaints systems might be misused to bully staff. Many Trusts do not even address the possibility that complaints could be vexatious ('instituted without sufficient grounds, especially so as to cause annoyance or embarrassment to the defendant': *Collins English Dictionary* 1994). Policies on aggression towards staff mostly limit themselves to severe verbal abuse and physical assault, whereas bullying often takes more subtle forms. The definition of bullying adopted by the DSPD unit mentioned earlier is: 'The use of strength or power to coerce or undermine others by fear'. It is important to acknowledge, in its application, that issues of dominance can be far from clear-cut, and that an apparently weaker party can find and use, very effectively, means of attack that are either inconspicuous or cloaked in an appearance of legitimacy.

Overtly 'psychopathic' patients are said to bully others for reasons of self-interest and lack of empathy (Cleckley 1941; Hare 1970). A study conducted as long ago as 1977, however, concluded that the concept of 'psychopath' was being used too widely and loosely (Gunn and Robertson 1977). In fact, most individuals with personality disorder do so in response to feelings of ill-treatment. The fact that difficulties in forming and maintaining relationships lie at the heart of the condition adds a great deal of complexity to the causes and meaning of this experience. There is no doubt that most of these individuals have suffered severe harm from an early age: family histories of psychological disturbance, multiple broken attachments (including periods in residential care), economic deprivation and social exclusion are common, while extremes of physical, sexual and emotional mistreatment have been experienced by 80 per cent of patients in forensic settings (Coid 1992). The sequelae of prolonged childhood abuse have been described as 'complex post-traumatic stress disorder' (Herman 1992). Features include poor regulation of emotions, alterations in consciousness such as depersonalisation and dissociation, difficulty with intimacy and identity confusion. Just as corrosive is the accompanying loss of a sense of agency and meaning in life (Livesley 2003).

A further consequence of childhood maltreatment is the phenomenon of 'identification with the aggressor' (Freud 1966; de Zulueta 1993; Norton 1996). An individual unconsciously repeats a traumatic experience in a way that makes *someone else* suffer the associated pain and humiliation. Thus he gains mastery over it, rather than being a powerless, passive recipient. An extreme sensitivity to the shame of victimhood also lies behind much serious violence: Gilligan (1996) has emphasised the great importance of using aggression as a means of 'getting respect'. This response to humiliation has been described by Fonagy and Target (2000): 'shame is felt as actually potentially annihilating – not an "as if" experience, but one where the psychological experience of mortification comes to be equated with the physical experience of destruction'. Thus, in adult life, many personality-disordered offenders carry out acts of physical or psychological violence when shamed, in order, as they perceive it, to preserve their very selves. Antisocial patients in particular attempt to control, deceive or use others, as ways of warding off the humiliation and cruelty they anticipate from others, and any failure in this effort increases the risk of aggression as a means of control.

Acts of harm to others can therefore be seen as a method of defending against inner subjectivity, or put more simply, painful thoughts and feelings, while the assumption of betrayal is built into the personality-disordered individual's experience of the 'other'. This has obvious, complex implications for complaints processes, which on the one hand can never 'resolve' a long-standing, grievous hurt, but on the other can provide a 'legitimate' vehicle for a re-enactment of the perpetrator role (Lowdell and Adshead 2009). Alternatively, the lodging of a complaint can be understood as a proxy for the pursuit of justice for wrongs experienced long ago: the sense of grievance and rage that childhood maltreatment engender are characteristically nurtured over time, and pursued relentlessly in the present day. Both the staff member complained about and the colleague(s) assigned to investigating and arbitrating the complaint can then become figures in the patient's own 'internal world drama' (Davies 1996), within a procedural frame that takes no account of this kind of transferential dynamic.

Personality-disordered individuals' propensity to perceive others as intending to cause them harm even when they do not has also been attributed to a failure of 'mentalization' (Bateman and Fonagy 2004), or an inability to 'read' correctly, and think about, the intentions of others. This can lead to one of the greatest difficulties for staff: these patients respond to care as though it were the abuse with which they are infinitely more familiar. Hinshelwood (2002) has described the vicious cycle that can ensue, with staff being rejected and denigrated for the very act of trying to offer help. In this way, the distorted interpretations of the intentions of others, and their emotional responses, contribute to personality-disordered patients' sometimes catastrophic interpersonal difficulties. It is particularly relevant for complaints processes that others are responded to as if they were abusive figures from the past – and thus inherently dangerous, cruel or exploitative. Of course, such is the long-standing stigma attached to the diagnosis of personality disorder (Lewis and Appleby 1988) that there are still many clinicians who, intentionally or otherwise, *do* cause harm via punitive responses and exclusion from services. These patients are exquisitely sensitive to deeply-held feelings of fear and dislike, which are often made manifest via an exercise of power far too subtle for any complaint by a 'psychopath' – or line management intervention – to be successful.

COMPLAINTS OF ILL-USAGE

To some extent, modern complaints systems provide personality-disordered offenders with an alternative to their previous criminal acts in the form of a pro-social means of seeking justice and respect. However, it will by now be obvious that these systems are open to misuse, and that this misuse is open to misunderstanding. In this section, I will illustrate how personality-disordered patients can consciously or unconsciously use complaints as a means of attack upon staff. It is crucial, however, not to interpret every instance of recourse to the formal complaints system as a *de facto* manifestation of psychopathology, or as always misguided.

As with most other secure forensic services in the NHS, the complaints process is explained to patients as soon as they arrive in the Unit, via Trust notices, posters and leaflets advertising the entitlement, and guaranteeing a response within twenty-five days. This practice immediately conveys an impression to both patients and clinicians, without it being stated explicitly, that investigating complaints about those offering care will be given priority over many other areas of legitimate concern, such as staffing levels, employees' complaints, the physical environment, and even treatment – one of the primary tasks of the organisation (Adshead 1998). Perhaps the only exception is a prominent sign proclaiming that 'Violence against staff will not be tolerated' – but such incidents are far less frequently examined (ironically, perhaps, because staff tend *not* to complain about them). Our Trust, like many others, defines a complaint as 'an event which the complainant wishes to be investigated by a person with the authority to take action and make changes, and which requires a response from the Chief Executive'. It will immediately be noted that the status of clinical authority is in question, and potentially put into the hands of management. Members of staff go about their daily work, therefore, with an awareness that the patient can potentially have their every action scrutinised by the Chief Executive, and that the patient knows it.

The Unit receives approximately one formal complaint per month; in practice, many months can pass without a complaint being lodged, and then several are made in quick succession, often by the same individual. It is the repeated and targeted use of complaints that alerts one to the possibility of a destructive, sadistic element to the intent behind them, and as with criminal acts, a few individuals are usually responsible for the vast majority of expressions of grievance. Recurring complaints against one individual often seem to be made with the desired effect of demeaning a member of staff in his or her professional role; perhaps this is no accident, role being a core source of identity, self-esteem and authority. The message being conveyed is that the staff member is an 'unfit' carer (Aiyegbusi 2009), in an echo of past experiences of failed care. Failed care leads to failed or insecure attachments, which are commonly associated with the expression of anger (Bowlby 1984), particularly towards care-givers (Main and George 1985).

Thus one patient began targeting a nurse by cornering him at the far end of the ward and venomously attacking the incompetence and bias he perceived in what the nurse had written in his notes. He expressed surprise and denials upon learning that he had reduced the nurse to tears, but went on to make a formal complaint when the same staff member was involved in a random search of his room. Other complaints followed, and while they were not upheld, the patient had succeeded in what seemed to the nurse to be the conscious goal of making him feel anxious, undermined and – rationally or not – fearful for his job. The patient had remarked, during the early days of his admission, that the nurse reminded him of the father who had threatened him with a loaded gun when he was six years old, by way of exerting discipline.

A different patient also attacked roles, recruiting his peers and making a particular target of students working in the Unit. This began with expressions of contempt for their relative lack of experience and qualifications, progressed to complaints if they attended clinical meetings, and finally ended with solicitors' letters to the Trust and the Nursing and Midwifery Council. In fact, NHS patients have the right not to have students involved in their care, and it seems that one of those involved had succeeded in getting them banned altogether from his previous secure institution. That this destructive achievement gave him a sense of power was undeniable. With some difficulty, a compromise was arrived at in the Unit that allowed the students to continue to work on the wards, but with restrictions in place. To be on the receiving end of such attacks early in one's career was, however, very demoralising. As another, uninvolved patient put it: 'Why would they (students) want to work with PD patients when they qualify, if this is how they get treated?' One of the patients involved had been attending university when he committed his index offence, which was sufficiently grave that he had never been able to resume his studies. It is perhaps interesting to speculate that students might represent all the promise and ambition of youth that has been denied these patients, and that the envious feelings thus aroused might be too painful to contemplate.

Patient complaints do provide opportunity for the Unit to learn from experience concerning good practice in the institutional response to the use of complaints as a tool for bullying. The treatment model is that of a modified therapeutic community (TC), about which more will be said later. There is an emphasis upon the value of openness, honesty and feedback from both peers and staff, particularly about offending behaviour. This brings its own challenges in an NHS setting: one patient formally complained that his confidentiality had been breached, after details of his particularly disturbing offence, an attack on a baby, were brought into a community meeting by a member of staff. Until then, the group had been aware only of the 'bare bones' of his conviction for attempted murder, due to our requirement for offence disclosure upon arrival in the Unit. The result of this more comprehensive revelation was a realistic fear of assault by his peers and an indelible experience of shame that led him to withdraw temporarily from treatment. The damage took time to contain and process, but we also wrote a protocol in collaboration with the patient group about confidentiality within community meetings. Honest self-scrutiny about the impact of our behaviour upon others is therefore required of staff, as well as of patients.

Some complaints are thus justifiable and deserving of an apology. This often goes a long way towards engaging patients in a more realistic treatment endeavour, in which the desire for perfect care gives way to a healthier acceptance of shortcomings. On other occasions the sense of having been wounded is hard to overcome. The patient mentioned above, whose offending was revealed in a community meeting, received both an apology and a copy of the confidentiality protocol we wrote as a result. But the 'forgiveness' of the member of staff took time: over a year later the patient made a further formal complaint about his technique when recording an electrocardiogram (ECG). This was an investigation the patient had himself requested, but he objected to the way the electrodes were attached. This complaint reached the Trust's medical director who, concerned about the exact technique that had been used, asked us to agree that any future tests should be performed by a clinician from outside the Unit if the patient so chose. The humiliation experienced by the member of staff was as complete as that originally felt by the patient – an example of projective identification in which the experience of public shaming in the community meeting was replicated and passed back to the 'shamer'. Thus the patient's unconsciously desired outcome of his complaint was achieved with the help of the 'system'. These were features of the entire exchange that the medical director, of course, could not be aware of.

ARE ALL COMPLAINTS EQUAL?
One difficulty with complaints processes is that all complaints are treated 'in good faith'. While on the face of it this approach is both neutral and fair, it ignores the possibility of complaints being vexatious, malicious, or even orchestrated. Thus a genuine commitment to making things better can become conflated with a stance that 'the customer is always right', or at least always has the right to complain. Even systems administered by mental health organisations can be oblivious to complaints that become an expression of ill-health, whether or not ill-usage has occurred. This is not always safe for staff. Thus one patient about whom our advice was sought had complained about deficiencies in her care in another part of the Trust, some of which were felt to be real. However, her insistence that she never again be treated in her home borough – on the grounds that none of the clinicians practising there could be trusted – was acceded to. Her contact with the complaints department then escalated to a torrent of increasingly aggressive voicemail messages, texts and e-mails. The

head of the complaints department, thinking to protect his colleagues while preserving the patient's right to complain, designated himself as her only point of contact. It was only when the patient threatened to kill his children, burn down Trust headquarters, and attack his staff with a machete as they came to work that a police escort was requested and criminal charges were finally brought against her. The patient was eventually diagnosed as suffering from a psychotic illness.

MANAGING COMPLAINTS IN CLINICAL PRACTICE

During the development of the Unit, which opened in 2005, we established two methods of thinking about and mitigating the damaging impact of complaints: first using the treatment model itself, and second through the provision of regular, protected time for reflective practice (see Chapters 13, 14 and 15 in this volume). Formal, written complaints are of course also dealt with via the established processes, being investigated either by a senior member of staff, or by a designated, independent person, depending upon the Trust's estimation of their severity.

Our chosen treatment model, a modified therapeutic community (TC) approach, has seen some success with severe personality disorder (Taylor 2000; Warren *et al*. 2003). Its core philosophy is to encourage a 'culture of enquiry' (Main 1946) via an open, collaborative and mutually respectful approach where questions can be asked (see also Chapters 1 and 8). The framework of three one-and-a-half-hour community meetings per week serves to provide opportunities for 'learning what feelings and perceptions lie behind behaviour, testing distorted perceptions against the common consensus' (Kennard 1998, p.61). Emotions and behaviours, in other words, have meaning and are important to try to understand. The community meetings provide a central platform to help these processes occur, by ensuring that all the interactions, events and activities taking place in the unit day and night are fed into a forum attended by all staff and patients. These include those inevitable difficulties and dissatisfactions that occur in all interpersonal relationships. Such experiences occur on a daily basis within the Unit, and often contribute greatly to our understanding of the patients' offending behaviour.

Thus when a complaint is made, the patient is encouraged to bring it to the community meeting for discussion, thus signifying to him that the whole community takes it seriously. He is helped to explore its meaning, both for him and for the staff member he has complained about, including why the staff member's action or lack of action induced such feelings of 'ill-usage'. A frequent and important theme to emerge is that of patients compartmentalising or splitting staff into 'all good', and 'all bad' camps; there are those who are idealised, and those who are denigrated and complained about (Klein 1975). Such divisions often, although not always, have little to do with real differences in attitude or behaviour. Since these patients can be highly insightful about each other's difficulties, peer feedback is often very successful at teasing out the origins of a negative transference, at reducing the pain of boundary setting, and at developing together a more integrated and reasonable view of the member of staff as a well-meaning but imperfect human being, working in an imperfect organisation. In a busy treatment unit situated within the bureaucratic and hierarchical structure of a hospital, small miscommunications, misunderstandings and misjudgements are inevitable. Committed clinicians, aware of the importance of achieving a therapeutic alliance, will often endeavour to right all these wrongs, even those that are not their responsibility. But in some ways the most important therapeutic task of all is to fail the patient, since shielding him from all the many shortfalls he might encounter in his life is unachievable. In keeping with Winnicott's description of the 'good enough mother' (1958), the task of treatment is in fact to 'dose' these failures, or to titrate them against what can be tolerated, such that omnipotence can gradually be relinquished and the capacity for concern developed. This task is, of course, at odds with a system designed to ensure that failures are 'investigated by a person with the authority to take action and make changes'.

There is an undeniable tension in the clinical team's dual role of conducting complaints procedures rigorously while also thinking critically about their meaning, and hopefully bringing that meaning into the whole group – patients and staff – for consideration. Such is the anxiety now generated by management in the face of some forms of external scrutiny – for example, unannounced visits by the Care Quality Commission – that these can have the paradoxical effect of encouraging the automatic rejection of complaints. Since these patients tend to subject care-givers to the same hatred they experienced as children (Higgit and Fonagy 1992), the experience of staff can be that of being criticised and found wanting in their roles from all sides. It is important, therefore, to provide less pressurised occasions for them to talk together about the painful feelings that are inevitably aroused: regular and frequent hand-overs, debriefs and reflective practice meetings give opportunities to understand how and why we often find ourselves forced into the position of the neglectful or abusive care-giver. This is crucial in order to promote thoughtful relational security and to limit unconscious acting out by staff, whether by 'defensive distancing' (Mackie 2009) or, worse, through punitive or vengeful practices. Even frequent multi-disciplinary reflection, however, does not always succeed in averting the sometimes malign inter-staff grievances (informal, formal and even anonymous) that so commonly arise – in a process paralleling the dynamic in the patients (Searles 1955) – within teams working with personality-disordered patients (Main 1957; see also Chapter 14).

It is important too for those complained about to be experienced by the patient as resilient in the face of his hatred: we have never, for example, changed a patient's primary nurse as a consequence of a complaint. In this way the patient learns that his nurse can survive his murderous projections. One patient, whose index offence was a violent sexual assault, had actually been slightly brain damaged after his father beat him repeatedly as a child. For over a year, this man was a serial complainer against his primary nurse, constantly accusing her of being 'unfit' for the job, and denigrating her in front of her colleagues. Such a message can be very difficult to hear, especially for staff who struggle with their own feelings of inadequacy for personal historical reasons, and who might therefore be inclined to fit in with this 'construct' of themselves (Neeld and Clarke 2009; see also Chapters 1 and 2). This individual was particularly sensitive to the language his nurse used in her reports about him, which did not gloss over the very provocative, even cruel, behaviour he sometimes engaged in on the ward. However, she was supported in her task of providing a consistent attachment figure, albeit one that did not shy away from confronting him with the reality of what he had become. He eventually came to understand this painful message, and to develop some capacity for concern for others. On his last day before transferring to another unit, the patient arranged a communal meal and read her a moving letter of thanks. This change was slow and partial, however, and positive new attachments remained difficult to form: we heard that, a week after arriving in his new placement, he had assaulted a staff member.

CONCLUSION

Formal complaints systems are an obligatory and necessary part of the way forensic mental health institutions ensure that their patients receive the best care. They are, however, open to misuse, especially by personality-disordered individuals who have highly toxic relationships with care-givers, being inclined to assign to them the roles their past abusers once occupied. It is essential that the meaning and impact of complaints is worked through therapeutically with patients, and that staff are helped to understand and process the highly negative projections they can represent. In many organisations, however, there is an unhelpful distance between clinicians and those managers (especially those without the benefit of a clinical background) who investigate complaints and attempt to 'put things right'. This can lead to staff feeling demoralised and undermined, while leaving the patient's sense of 'ill-treatment' unresolved. Ways need to be found, perhaps through joint training and learning from examples, of making such systems more integrated without losing their independence and the capacity to respond effectively to real instances of poor practice.

REFERENCES

Adshead, G. (1998) 'Psychiatric staff as attachment figures: understanding management problems in psychiatric services in the light of attachment theory.' *British Journal of Psychiatry 172*, 64–89.

Aiyegbusi, A. (2009) 'The Nurse-Patient Relationship with Offenders: Containing the Unthinkable to Promote Recovery.' In A. Aiyegbusi and J. Clarke-Moore (eds) *Therapeutic Relationships with Offenders: An Introduction to the Psychodynamics of Forensic Mental Health Nursing*. London: Jessica Kingsley Publishers.

Bateman, A. and Fonagy, P. (2004) *Psychotherapy for Borderline Personality Disorder: Mentalization-Based Treatment*. Oxford: Oxford University Press.

Bowlby, J. (1984) 'Violence in the family as a disorder of the attachment and care-giving systems.' *American Journal of Psychoanalysis 44*, 9–27.

Cleckley, H. (1941) *The Mask of Sanity* (5th Edition). Augusta, Georgia: Emily S. Cleckley.

Coid, J. (1992) 'DSM-II diagnoses in criminal psychopaths; the way forward.' *Criminal Behaviour and Mental Health 2*, 78–95.

Collins English Dictionary (1994) Glasgow: HarperCollins Publishers.

Criminal Justice Act (2003) London: HMSO.

Davies, R. (1996) 'The Interdisciplinary Network and the Internal World of the Offender.' In C. Cordess and M. Cox (eds) *Forensic Psychotherapy: Crime, Psychodynamics and the Offender Patient*. London: Jessica Kingsley Publishers.

Department of Health (1992) *Committee of Inquiry into Complaints about Ashworth Hospital*. London: HMSO.

Department of Health (1999) *Report of the Committee of Inquiry into the Personality Disorder Unit, Ashworth Special Hospital.* London: Department of Health.

Department of Health (2000) *A Plan for Investment, a Plan for Reform.* London: Department of Health.

Department of Health (2010) *The NHS Constitution for England.* London: Department of Health.

de Zulueta, F. (1993) *From Pain to Violence: The Traumatic Roots of Destructiveness.* London: Whurr Publishers.

Fonagy, P. and Target, M. (2000) 'Attachment and reflective function: Their role in self-organisation.' *Developmental Psychopathology 9*, 679–700.

Freud, A. (1966) *The Ego and the Mechanisms of Defence.* London: The Hogarth Press and the Institute of Psychoanalysis.

Gilligan, J. (1996) *Reflections on Our Deadliest Epidemic.* London: Jessica Kingsley Publishers.

Gunn, J. and Robertson, G. (1977) 'Psychopathic personality: a conceptual problem.' *Psychological Medicine 6*, 631–634.

Hare, R. (1970) *Psychopathy: Theory and Research.* New York: Wiley.

Herman, J. (1992) *Trauma and Recovery.* New York: Basic Books.

Higgit, A. and Fonagy, P. (1992) 'Psychotherapy in borderline and narcissistic personality disorder.' *British Journal of Psychiatry 161*, 23–43.

Hinshelwood, R.D. (2002) 'Abusive help – helping abuse: the psychodynamic impact of severe personality disorder on caring institutions.' *Criminal Behaviour and Mental Health 12*, S20–S30.

Kennard, D. (1998) *An Introduction to Therapeutic Communities.* London: Jessica Kingsley Publishers.

Klein, M. (1975) *Envy and Gratitude.* London: The Hogarth Press and the Institute of Psychoanalysis.

Lester, G., Wilson, B., Griffin, L. and Mullen, P. (2004) 'Unusually persistent complainants.' *British Journal of Psychiatry 184*, 352–356.

Lewis, G. and Appleby, L. (1988) 'Personality disorder: the patients psychiatrists dislike.' *British Journal of Psychiatry 153*, 44–49.

Liveseley, J. (2003) *Practical Management of Personality Disorder.* New York: The Guilford Press.

Lowdell, A. and Adshead, G. (2009) 'The Best Defence: Institutional Defences Against Anxiety in Forensic Services.' In A. Aiyegbusi and J. Clarke-Moore (eds) *Therapeutic Relationships with Offenders: An Introduction to the Psychodynamics of Forensic Mental Health Nursing.* London: Jessica Kingsley Publishers.

Mackie, S. (2009) 'Reflecting on Murderousness: Reflective Practice in Secure Forensic Settings.' In A. Aiyegbusi and J. Clarke-Moore (eds) *Therapeutic Relationships with Offenders: An Introduction to the Psychodynamics of Forensic Mental Health Nursing.* London: Jessica Kingsley Publishers.

Main, T. (1946) 'The Hospital as Therapeutic Institution.' *Bulletin of the Menninger Clinic 10*, 66–70.

Main, T. (1957) 'The ailment.' *British Journal of Medical Psychology 30*, 3, 129–145.

Main, M. and George, C. 1985) 'Responses of abused and disadvantaged toddlers to distress in age-mates: a study in a day care setting.' *Developmental Psychology 21*, 407–412.

National Institute for Mental Health in England (2003) *The Personality Disorder Capabilities Framework*. London: Department of Health.

Neeld, R. and Clarke, T. (2009) 'The Patient, Her Nurse and the Therapeutic Community.' In A. Aiyegbusi and J. Clarke-Moore (eds) *Therapeutic Relationships with Offenders: An Introduction to the Psychodynamics of Forensic Mental Health Nursing*. London: Jessica Kingsley Publishers.

NHS Choices (2008) *NHS Choices: Delivering for the NHS*. London: Department of Health.

Norton, K. (1996) 'The Personality-Disordered Forensic Patient and the Therapeutic Community.' In C. Cordess and M. Cox (eds) *Forensic Psychotherapy: Crime, Psychodynamics and the Offender Patient. Vol II: Mainly Practice*. London: Jessica Kingsley Publishers.

Searles, H. (1955) 'The informational value of the supervisor's emotional experience.' *Psychiatry 18*, 135–146.

Shaw, J., Davies, J. and Morey, H. (2001) 'An assessment of the security, dependency and treatment needs of all patients in secure services in a UK health region.' *Journal of Forensic Psychiatry and Psychology 12*, 610–637.

Taylor, C. (2011) 'Nothing left to lose? Freedom and compulsion in the treatment of dangerous offenders.' *Psychodynamic Practice 17*, 3, 291–306.

Taylor, R. (2000) *A Seven Year Reconviction Study of HMP Grendon Therapeutic Community*. Research Findings 115. London: Home Office Research, Development and Statistics Directorate.

Warren, F., Preedy, K., McGauley, G. *et al.* (2003) *Review of Treatments for Dangerous and Severe Personality Disorder*. London: Department of Health.

Winnicott, D.W. (1958) *Collected Papers*. London: Tavistock Publications.

Chapter 5

YOUR FRIENDS AND NEIGHBOURS
Professional Boundary Violations – A Review of
Perpetrator Typologies and Impact on Clients

Jonathan Coe

*In this chapter Jonathan Coe explores the minefield of attacks upon the
therapeutic milieu from would-be helpers. He compares and contrasts typologies
of professionals who abuse their patients in a range of different settings. In such
cases, perhaps in contrast to Taylor's account in the previous chapter, complaints
systems may in fact be* under-used, *for fear of betrayal on the part of the patient,
or because the professional has convinced them that the violation was justified,
deserved, or even solicited. In these cases the very foundation of therapeutic work,
personal and professional integrity, has been undermined. He refers to the recent
collapse of the initiative to establish statutory regulation of the profession of
psychotherapy, so the reader is left to wonder if there is a societal over-investment
in protecting privatised interests, typified by a therapeutic preoccupation with
privileging one-to-one helping relationships. Coe explores in detail the impact
of boundary violations upon the patient and builds upon a wealth of experience
working with the perpetrators of such violations in order to develop suggestions
for intervention with the system of care as a whole to address this pernicious
problem.*

INTRODUCTION

> I had no intentions of hurting him. [...] Mr. Jackson was my friend. I
> loved him. We had a great relationship. I was there to help him and I
> was going to be available should something go wrong, to help provide
> the best care for him. (Dr Conrad Murray in LAPD 2009)

Intrusions into the therapeutic space may originate from the practitioner,
the client or from external forces, but what they have in common is
that it is always the practitioner's responsibility to maintain professional
boundaries, or to reset them as necessary. Was Dr Murray cynically

using the notion of friendship with Michael Jackson as an attempt at exculpation, or was the socialisation of their relationship a material precursor for professional misconduct? As Gabbard (2011) has said, 'Practitioners have codes of conduct and ethics to abide by, clients do not.'

This chapter is concerned with the responsibilities of the practitioner and looks at how the perpetrators of boundary violations have been categorised by previous writers and practitioners, as well as accounting for the ways in which clients may be harmed as a result of practitioner action.

Whilst much of the literature base on professional boundaries is from psychology and psychotherapy, the issues are relevant for all disciplines which have a fiduciary responsibility towards those using their services. My central argument is that an understanding of the modes of behaviour of transgressing professionals, and of the impact on clients, are important, but that this focus needs to be accompanied by a radically increased awareness of the potential of all practitioners to transgress; and that this is vital if we are to make significant inroads into the ultimate aim of reducing harm and minimising transgressions. It is how we behave, rather than who we are, that is determinative.

Serious violations of professional boundaries are of critical relevance for all practitioners and for everyone who uses their services: all may become violator or victim.

PROFESSIONAL BOUNDARIES

Gabbard and Lester (1995) describe boundaries by use of a reifying metaphor: 'Visitors to the Grand Canyon note that they are protected from falling into the chasm by a guardrail placed strategically at the edge of the canyon. This safety measure allows children (and adults) to play and enjoy themselves while being at minimal risk for catastrophe. Although analytic boundaries in general are more flexible than a guardrail, in some areas, such as sexual contact, they are just as unyielding' (p.59). They summarise professional boundaries as 'a set of behaviours concerning: role; time; place and space; money; gifts; services; clothing; language; self-disclosure; and physical contact.' Marilyn Peterson has identified boundaries as 'the limits that allow for a safe connection based on the client's needs' (Peterson 1992). Andrea Celenza provides a nuanced description of boundaries in professional practice:

The creation of boundaries is at once a psychic necessity and an illusion. The need to draw lines allows for the existence of categories – this is this and not that – and, in this way, boundaries make thinking possible. We also establish rules that demarcate psychic space: don't touch me there, don't ask me that. However, there are no real lines, even on a physical level, just horizons where one entity meets another and the outer skin defines the borders between the two. In the psychic world, the lines are more blurry still. Who is to say where one's self ends and the other begins?

The boundary demarcating two separate existences is a needed perceptual differentiation in order that our thoughts and feelings may be categorized and felt as me-not-you. Thus, it is through boundaries that the self is born. Yet, in relationships, as in analysis, these psychic boundaries are invisible, and the distinction of one's self as different and separate from another must be asserted and reasserted in a continuous and ongoing way. (Celenza 2007a, p.xiii)

The author Ursula Le Guin (1974) adds another useful dimension in her utopian novel *The Dispossessed*: '[The wall] degenerated into mere geometry, a line, an idea of boundary. But the idea was real. It was important. [...] Like all walls it was ambiguous, two-faced. What was inside it and what was outside it depended upon which side of it you were on' (p.9).

It follows that violations of these boundaries may lead to catastrophe but paradoxically may also be hard to see clearly, especially during the early stages (Russell 1993). Violations go significantly beyond the sexual and can include: encouraging dependency through misdiagnosis; forming business relationships with clients; exploiting clients for financial gain; excessive self-disclosure; belittling/demeaning; pathologising; failing to treat; working beyond competence; breaking confidentiality; encouraging idealising transferences; abrupt termination of treatment; reversing roles; discussing other patients; taking phone calls/answering emails in session.

PREVALENCE AND REGULATION

There has been no definitive study of the prevalence of professional misconduct issues in the UK (Garrett 2010). The prevalence of sexual boundary violations has been difficult to determine as there have been relatively few studies and those that have taken place have adopted differing methodologies (Pope 2001). The inquiry into the psychiatrists Kerr and Haslam suggested that, on the limited available research evidence, between 3 and 6 per cent of UK doctors may have had sexual contact with one or more of their patients, producing what the inquiry describes as the 'startling statistical interpolation' of 6500 to 13,000 doctors (Pleming 2005, p.621). Subotsky notes that sexual misconduct was the major issue for professional misconduct hearings at the General Medical Council (GMC) for psychiatrists in the period she studied (Subotsky 2010). The only research survey in the UK was undertaken by Garrett (Garrett 1994) with 1000 clinical psychologists (58% response rate); this study's main finding was that 22.7 per cent of those surveyed had treated patients who had been sexually involved with previous therapists. The best review of previous prevalence surveys was carried out by Pope (2001) in the USA. He pooled data from eight national peer-reviewed self-report studies of therapists. He found a prevalence rate for sexual contact between therapists and clients of seven per cent of male therapists, 1.5 per cent of female therapists, giving an average of 4.4 per cent of therapists. Some indications are provided by the published data from the statutory health regulators, summarised by the Council for Healthcare Regulatory Excellence (CHRE). Their figures for all regulators show that in a five-year period there were 325 'sexual misconduct' cases investigated and 199 cases concerning 'failure to maintain appropriate professional boundaries'.[1] CHRE's 'Clear Sexual Boundaries' project (Stone, Halter and Brown 2007) research found that between 38 per cent and 52 per cent of health professionals report knowing of colleagues who have been sexually involved with patients. The GMC investigated 218 allegations of 'improper relationships with patients' about 169 doctors over a one year period.[2] Unfortunately there is little information available from self-regulatory organisations for counselling and psychotherapy or from occupations such as complementary therapies.

Professional regulators such as the GMC have a range of sanctions available to them, typically including issuing a warning; agreeing undertakings; imposing conditions of practice or suspension; and erasure from the register. Adjudication panels typically have a three-part process: 1) the determination on facts; 2) whether these amount to an impaired fitness to practice; 3) sanction. Sanctions in particular

---

1   Email communication with the author April 2010.
2   Email communication with the author March 2010.

cases may be affected by mitigating factors (such as levels of remorse and insight, remediation) and aggravating factors (such as exploitation of the patient). Self-regulators (usually professional associations) have very diverse processes, standards and responses, which are not always transparent and which are not easily summarised here. Sanctions in practice range from 'no case to answer', through the requirement to write an essay, to removal from the register. There has been no systematic cross-professional review of conduct decisions related to boundary violations.

PERPETRATORS

The danger of reviewing published typologies of transgressive practitioners is that practitioners may be encouraged to feel that colleagues who violate boundaries are somehow divorced from the rest of the professional field. Gabbard says, 'I'm convinced that people hate complexity – they like to say "all of these guys are bad, they're evil, they're predators, let's throw them out, throw the bad apple out of the barrel, then everything will be fine"' (Coe 2010), adding that, 'This allows us to disown our own vulnerability' (Gabbard 2011). Totton (2001) has described the wish to expel aberrant practitioners from the profession as 'a chronic fantasy that we can get rid of all the messy, dirty, chaotic aspects of therapy and counselling.' Developing a nuanced understanding of how transgressions come about will be vital for anyone interested in the possibility of rehabilitation.

The experience of expert evaluators of transgressing professionals is that there are significant numbers of perpetrators who have led otherwise unblemished professional lives who then commit some kind of serious misconduct (Gabbard 2011). The line between the 'good' practitioner and the 'bad' is very fine and in fact Gabbard argues that it is largely illusory (ibid). He posits that in this regard the superego is best seen as fluid rather than as a 'fixed point containing holes' (ibid). This analysis helps us to see aberrant behaviour as grounded in 'normal' practitioners rather than simply in a small contained group of predators.

There are of course some well-known examples of predatory practitioners who exploit large numbers of vulnerable clients over many years. In the UK there have been at least 22 proven cases of serial sexual exploitation by doctors (internet review 2011) since the turn of the century (involving criminal prosecutions or cases proven at the GMC). There have been at least five major public inquiries into this kind of abuse (Pleming 2005; Pauffley 2004; McKenna and Hussain 2004; Limbach and Hopkins 2009; Commission for Health Improvement 2001) and an unknown number of internal management reviews in the NHS. Whilst these cases dominate the headlines and have influenced some significant policy changes at a national level[3] the extent of boundary violations affecting single clients remains unknown.

TYPOLOGIES

Work to consider what measures should be in place to improve public protection and to assess the relevance of rehabilitation measures is now gradually being explored in the UK (Coe 2010b; Snowden 2010). In this context it may be helpful to consider how specialists have articulated their clinical findings concerning the character of practitioners who have transgressed boundaries.

Devereux (2011) has identified four discrete conceptual categories which describe the *types of behaviour* which are mobilised by practitioner in harmful therapy. Devereux undertook a grounded theory analysis of published client accounts of harmful therapy which resulted in the identification of four types of problematic behaviour:

- misusing professional knowledge
- exploiting the therapeutic process
- perverting the therapy
- depriving the client of the therapeutic space.

From this Devereux identified the core category of 'using the client instrumentally' or 'objectification' of the client. Devereux states that 'this was resonant with Kant's core ethical principle [...] which proposes that the locus of the unethical is in the use of a subject merely as a means to an end.'

Schoener and Gonsiorek (1989) describe six categories which they tag as 'diagnostic':

1. uninformed/naïve
2. healthy or mildly neurotic
3. severely neurotic and/or socially isolated
4. impulsive character disorders

---

3   For example, the Clear Boundaries Project, published by the CHRE 2008.

5. sociopathic or narcissistic character disorders

6. psychotic or borderline personalities.

They added a seventh in 1994:

7. bipolar disorders.

Schoener[4] says of these that 'the categories were originally created [...] as a way of responding to victim questions such as "why did this happen?" or "why did he do this?" They proved useful in working with ethics committees, licensing boards, employers and others. At the time we created them in the late 1970s to the degree that anyone paid attention to the "why" question, they tended to have over-simplified views. Many saw this as a problem which just required a bit of therapy, whereas others believed that people could not be rehabilitated. We tried, and I think succeeded, in helping change the conversation from punishment to rehabilitation.' He adds: 'We have never used the categories as a sorting or classification mechanism. Most people did not fit neatly into one or the other.'

Irons (1995, pp.163–175) presents a set of 'archetypal categories', based on assessments of practitioners undergoing inpatient treatment and heavily influenced by an approach to rehabilitation based on addiction theory:

- *The naïve prince*: early in career, feels invulnerable, tends to develop 'special relationships' with certain types of clients and blurs boundaries.

- *The wounded warrior*: overwhelmed by demands, overly dependent on professional mantle for validation; patient involvement; temporary escape.

- *The self-serving martyr*: middle or late career; work is primary; withdrawn, angry, and resentful.

- *The false lover*: enjoys living on the edge, the 'thrill of the chase'; a risk-taker who desires adventure.

- *The dark king*: powerful and charming; successful, manipulative; sexual exploitation as an expression of power.

- *The wild card*: erratic course in personal and professional life; significant difficulties in functioning; has major Axis I disorder.

---

4   Personal communication with the author November 2011.

Gabbard articulated what he describes as a 'psycho-dynamically based typology of analysts who have transgressed sexual boundaries', based on the experience of assessing and treating 70 cases of therapists who had sex with their patients (Gabbard and Lester 1995, p.92). He stresses that the categories 'should not be excessively reified or viewed as having rigid demarcations. Some practitioners have features of more than one category, and occasionally an idiosyncratic clinician may defy inclusion in any of these categories' (ibid, p.93). The four categories are:

1. psychotic disorders

2. predatory psychopathy and paraphilias

3. lovesickness

4. masochistic surrender.

Gabbard comments that the category of psychotic disorders is very rare but that the category encompassing psychopathy and the paraphilias is more common than generally supposed. He states that '[...] therapists in this category regard patients as objects to be used for their own gratification. Because they lack empathy or concern for the victim, they are largely incapable of feeling remorse or guilt about any harm they may have done to the patient' (ibid, p.95). He also notes that practitioners more advanced in their careers and often well respected are high risk: 'I have so many examples of that – the narcissistic guy who's well known in the field who says "Well you know the rules don't really apply to me anymore, because I know what I'm doing. If one of my supervisees did this I'd be worried about it, but I know what I'm doing, so I can get away with it". It's crazy but that's one of the rationalisations' (Coe 2010a).

Gabbard asserts that 'lovesickness' accounts for the majority of sexually transgressing analysts. The practitioner claims that the transgression was 'true love', has nothing to do with transference and is somehow outside the power differential inherent in professional relationships. 'When the analyst is male, the typical scenario is that a middle-aged practitioner falls madly in love with a much younger female patient. This infatuation usually occurs in the context of extreme stress in the analyst's life. The stressors may include divorce, separation, illness in a child or spouse, death of a family member, or disillusionment with his own marriage or career' (Gabbard and Lester 1995, p.96).

Masochistic surrender refers to the passive-aggressive clinician who goes along with client demands, says Gabbard: 'These therapists appear to pursue humiliation and victimization in their work and often in their private lives as well. [...] These clinicians characteristically have problems dealing with their own aggression. To assert their own rights or to set limits on the patient is viewed as cruel and sadistic, so all anger is turned inward in the form of self-defeating behaviours and attitudes' (ibid, p.113).

Pope and Bouhoutsos (1986) identified ten 'common scenarios of therapist-patient sexual intimacy'. The following are scenarios rather than diagnostic categories and were developed from the writers' own clinical experience, the clinical and research literature and public records.

- *Role trading.* Therapist becomes the 'patient' and the wants and needs of the therapist become the focus.

- *Sex therapy.* Therapist-patient sexual intimacy is presented as a valid treatment.

- *As if...* Positive transference treated as if it were not the result of the therapeutic situation.

- *Svengali.* Creation and exploitation of an exaggerated dependence.

- *Drugs.* Use of drugs as part of seduction.

- *Rape.* Physical force, threats or intimidation used.

- *True love.* Therapeutic situation is ignored through rationalisations.

- *It just got out of hand.* Emotional closeness of therapy not respected.

- *Time out.* Meetings outside the consulting room treated as though separate from the therapeutic relationship.

- *Hold me.* Exploitation of the patient's desire for non-erotic physical contact.

Like Schoener and Gabbard, Pope and Bouhoutsos also emphasise that there are exceptions to the categories and that each case has 'its own dynamics and likely course of development' and that 'each of the patients and therapists [the scenarios] experience this destructive event in his or her own way in the context of his or her unique life.'

Andrea Celenza, who has specialised in treating boundary-violating psychotherapists, identified the following characteristics from her study of 50 cases of sexual misconduct by therapists, which are described as precursors of, and risk factors for, therapist-patient sexual misconduct (2007b, pp.29–38). Celenza ties this list to the narcissistic, needy, lovesick or masochistic surrender types:

1. narcissistic vulnerability of long-standing

2. grandiose (covert) rescue fantasies

3. intolerance of negative transference

4. childhood history of emotional deprivation and sexualised over-stimulation

5. family history of covert and sanctioned boundary transgressions

6. unresolved anger toward authority figures

7. restricted awareness of fantasy (especially hostile/aggressive)

8. transformation of countertransference hate to countertransference love.

Understanding that these characteristics are likely to be present in this group may give clinicians charged with remedial treatment a head start in terms of noticing what their clients bring – the list can act as a checklist for the treatment of offending clinicians.

PEOPLE WHO HAVE BEEN VICTIMISED, NOT 'VICTIMS'

Who are the 'victims' of professional boundary violations? To the extent that there has been any public dialogue about the abuse by professionals of adult clients the assumption has often been that people who have been wounded in this way are exceptionally vulnerable, with histories of abuse, challenging or seductive behaviours, borderline traits or heightened passivity. In my experience practitioners defending allegations of abuse will often retrospectively diagnose clients as personality disordered, as a tactic intended to discredit the complaint. This can backfire on the practitioner as, if there is evidence of personality disorder, this would and should have been recorded and discussed with a supervisor and of course therapists working with people diagnosed with personality disorders need to take more care when managing boundaries, rather than less (Lion 1999).

Now, vulnerability is an issue and of course it is true that people who are less able to speak up for themselves are inherently more vulnerable to unwanted attention. High profile cases extensively reported on by mainstream media often do involve particularly vulnerable groups exploited by practitioners without remorse or concern for the harm they cause. Nurse manager David Britten targeted up to 60 young women suffering from eating disorders requiring inpatient treatment; psychiatrists Kerr and Haslam targeted emotionally vulnerable and isolated young women; East London GP Healy sexually abused under-age boys. The 2011 Panorama investigation of Castlebeck care home concerned the physical abuse of people with learning disabilities, while young children were once again the subjects of abuse at the Ealing Church inquiry report of 2011.

Professional groups opposing statutory regulation for counselling and psychotherapy have asserted that normal categories of abuse do not apply to the field, and that problems in psychotherapy arise from the misapplied feelings of the client who is challenged by the process of therapy, or transference. However, the overall focus on vulnerability in my view is also informed by a basic fear – that we are not as invulnerable as we think. We inherently want to believe that 'this couldn't happen to me' or 'I would never let this happen to me' – that it is something for people 'over there', the 'vulnerable', the 'mentally ill', the 'victims', the 'disordered' (Coe 2008).

As others have written (Gabbard and Gabbard 1999), cinematic portrayals often confirm these assumptions, with patients shown as stalkers (as in *What About Bob?*) or seductresses (as in *Final Analysis*) and practitioners as genuinely 'in love' with the patient (*Lovesick, Mr Jones*), healing them with their transformative 'love' (*The Prince of Tides*) – or 'victims' themselves of overbearing and loveless rules and authorities (*Don Juan De Carlo*). In fact, people from all economic, social and intellectual backgrounds have been subject to violations of professional boundaries and this is evidenced both from the published client literature and from the experience of specialist support agencies (Devereux 2010).

IMPACT

Effects of abuse will vary with the nature and severity of transgressions, and according to the background and level of vulnerability of the client involved. The harm caused can range from temporary emotional upset to longer-term trauma, including self-harming or suicidal behaviours. Devereux has described the notion of 'adverse idealising transference' in relation to boundary transgressions (2010). She has described the following impacts associated with boundary violations such as excessive disclosure:

- *Idealisation.* The therapist's status and asymmetrical knowledge base provide fertile ground for idealization to be established.

- *Elation.* The patient experiences an overwhelming feeling of elation as a result of being so important and special to such an exalted and idealised person.

- *Transcendence.* The feeling of elation has a transcendent effect that appears to make the problems that brought the client into therapy disappear.

- *Bonding.* Because the transcendence is so closely related to the person of the therapist the patient becomes bonded to the therapist and is then compelled to maintain the relationship at all costs.

- *Dependency.* The therapist quite literally becomes more important to the client than anything else in life. This makes the pain of being simply 'a client' unbearable. This means that the client will look for ways in which the relationship can become more 'real', leading in many cases to a sexual relationship.

The violation of professional boundaries may have serious and long-lasting psychological effects on the client, which may require intensive remedial attention. Pope and Bouhoutsos (1986) identified the following as commonly occurring:

- ambivalence

- anger

- guilt

- depression and suicide risk

- isolation

- sexual confusion

- cognitive dysfunction.

From the experience of working with survivors of boundary violations can be added:

- sense of humiliation or shame
- impaired ability to trust in any relationship
- inability to trust own judgement
- post-traumatic stress disorder type symptoms
- loss of self-esteem and loss of confidence
- extreme distress, including unresolved grief
- self-harming behaviours
- anxiety.

In addition, there is the vicious cycle of:

- failure to have the original problems (for which help was sought) dealt with
- worsening of the original problems
- impaired ability to approach or trust treating professionals
- additional damage inflicted by the abuse.

There are many parallels in the effects of sexual abuse by a health or care professional with the effects of childhood sexual abuse, and with domestic violence and sexual crimes in general. Self-blame is common. Clients may begin to rely on a range of defence mechanisms to protect them from acknowledging the violation that has occurred. In particular, it may be many years before they are able to recognise what happened and/or to take steps to deal with it.

The professional typically erodes the professional boundaries gradually and starts going down a 'slippery slope' (Simon 1995):

- gradual erosion of professional neutrality
- boundary violations begin 'between the chair and the door'
- socialisation of sessions
- client is treated as 'special'
- disclosure of confidential information about other clients

- professional begins making self-disclosures
- physical contact begins (e.g. touching, hugs, kisses)
- professional gains control over client
- contact occurs outside of sessions
- sessions extended in time
- sessions rescheduled for end of day
- professional stops billing client
- dating begins
- professional-client sex begins.

Following these experiences clients often experience significant blocks to validation and healing:

- Shame and secrecy, plus invisibility of psychological wounds, mean that clients question the validity of their own experiences.
- Lack of understanding from friends, family or professionals.
- May be inaccurately diagnosed as borderline, paranoid, or having an anxiety disorder.
- Unavailability of appropriate care or support.
- Services may be withdrawn by other health and care professionals.
- Feeling belittled, trivialised, blamed during court or complaints process. Lack of support or even secondary victimisation by friends and family.
- Losses suffered during and after the abuse – marriage, children, savings, job or career, house, health.
- A persistent lack of confidence, shame, self-blame and difficulty trusting their judgement of people and situations.
- Feeling in limbo, unable to progress with their lives, frequently re-traumatised during court or complaints process.

There may also be profound destructive effects on the family and others close to the abused client. Pope and Vetter's research (1990) found that harm occurred for about 90 per cent of patients who engaged in therapist-patient sex; harm occurred for about 80 per cent when the sex began only after termination; 11 per cent required hospitalisation of the patient; 14 per cent involved patient suicide attempts; 1 per cent involved completed suicides; and only 12 per cent involved formal complaints.

CONCLUSION

This short account of issues relating both to those who transgress and to those affected by transgressions is part of an ongoing attempt to place the majority of such behaviours firmly in the realm of the ordinary practice of ordinary practitioners. The key points, about the universality of risk and transgression, have been made before, notably by Schoener and Gabbard. This focus has been difficult to maintain, in part because of an ongoing professional reticence about misconduct, in part because of a lack of sustained and informed public attention and in part because of the stop-start nature of national policy developments relating to regulation.

Power differentials, setting, therapeutic process, boundary awareness and assumptions about healing are key and deserve wide attention as, given the 'right' set of circumstances, all practitioners may become violators and everyone who uses services has the potential of being victimised. Education of both practitioners and the public is a key factor in endeavours to manage and to minimise risk in this domain. Some of the central themes to be emphasised are:

- Understanding the power differential – including access to private information, knowledge, statutory roles.

- Setting – may be one-to-one, private practice, minimal external scrutiny.

- Process – therapeutic process involves being vulnerable, sharing intimate information, with the possibility of mishandling transferential and counter-transferential feelings.

- Commitment to the need for ongoing supervision and mentoring.

- Openness – willing to be accountable.

REFERENCES

Celenza, A. (2007a) 'Foreword.' In I. Kogan, *Escape from Selfhood: Breaking Boundaries and Craving for Oneness*. London: Karnac.

Celenza, A. (2007b) *Sexual Boundary Violations – Therapeutic, Supervisory and Academic Contexts*. New York: Aronson.

Coe, J. (2008) 'Preface.' In S. Richardson and M. Cunningham, *Broken Boundaries: Stories of Betrayal in Relationships of Care*. London: WITNESS.

Coe, J. (2010a) 'Boundary Violations – Our Friends and Colleagues: An Interview with Glen Gabbard.' *New Associations*. Available at www.psychoanalytic-council. org/main/index.php?page=154968, accessed on 24 January 2012.

Coe, J. (2010b) *USA Responses To Professional Boundary Violations*. London: Winston Churchill Memorial Trust.

Commission for Health Improvement (2001) *Investigation into issues arising from the case of Loughborough GP Peter Green*. London: The Stationery Office.

Devereux, D. (2010) *Ethics in Principle and Practice: The Client's Experience of Psychotherapy*. University of Kent.

Gabbard, G. (2011) 'Ethics, Self-Deception and the Corrupt Physician.' 28th Edward Glover Lecture. Unpublished conference paper.

Gabbard, G. and Lester, E. (1995) *Boundaries and Boundary Violations in Psychoanalysis*.: American Psychiatric Publishing Inc.

Gabbard, K. and Gabbard, G. (1999) *Psychiatry and the Cinema*. American Psychiatric Press.

Garrett, T. (1994) 'Epidemiology in the UK.' In D. Jehu (ed.) *Patients as Victims: Sexual Abuse in Psychotherapy and Counselling*. London: Wiley.

Garrett, T. (2010) 'The Prevalence of Boundary Violations Between Mental Health Practitioners and their Clients.' In F. Subotsky, S. Bewley and M. Crowe (eds) *Abuse of the Doctor-Patient Relationship*. London: RCPsych.

Irons, R. (1995) 'An Inpatient Assessment Model for Offenders.' In J. Gonsiorek (ed.) *Breach of Trust: Sexual Exploitation by Health Care Professionals and Clergy*. Thousand Oaks, CA: Sage.

LAPD (2009) *Transcript of recorded interview of Conrad Murray*. Los Angeles: Los Angeles Police Department Internal Affairs Group.

Le Guin, U. (1974) *The Dispossessed*. New York: Harper & Row.

Limbach, H. and Hopkins, S. (2009) *External review into the case of Roy Murray*. Manchester: NHS North-West.

Lion, J. (1999) 'Countertransference in the Treatment of the Antisocial Patient.' In G. Gabbard (ed.) *Countertransference Issues in Psychiatric Treatment*. Washington, DC: American Psychiatric Press.

McKenna, A. and Hussain, T. (2004) An Independent Investigation into the Conduct of David Britten at the Peter Dally Clinic. London: Verita.

Pauffley, T. (2004) Independent Investigation Into How the NHS Handled Allegations About The Conduct Of Clifford Ayling. London: HMSO.

Peterson, M. (1992) At Personal Risk: Boundary Violations in Professional-Client Relationships. New York: Norton.

Pleming, N. (2005) The Kerr/Haslam Inquiry. London: HMSO.

Pope, K. (2001) 'Sex Between Therapists and Clients.' In J. Worell (ed.) *Encyclopedia of Women and Gender: Sex Similarities and Differences and the Impact of Society on Gender*. New York: Academic Press.

Pope, K. and Bouhoutsos, J. (1986) *Sexual Intimacy Between Therapists and Patients*. Westport: Praeger.

Pope, K. and Vetter, V. (1990) 'Prior therapist-patient sexual involvement among patients seen by psychologists.' *Psychotherapy 28*, 3, 429–438.

Russell, J. (1993) Out of Bounds – Sexual Exploitation in Counselling and Psychotherapy. London: Sage.

Schoener, G. and Gonsiorek, J. (1989) 'Assessment & Development of Rehabilitation Plans for the Therapist. In Psychotherapists' Sexual Involvement with their Clients: Intervention & Prevention, Ch 32. Minneapolis: Walk-In Counselling Center.

Simon, R. (1995) 'The natural history of therapist sexual misconduct: identification and prevention.' *Psychiatric Annals 25*, 2, 90–94.

Snowden, P. (2010) 'Dealing with Offending Doctors: Sanctions and Remediation.' In F. Subotsky, S. Bewley and M. Crowe (eds) *Abuse of the Doctor-Patient Relationship*. London: RCPsych Publications.

Stone, J., Halter, M. and Brown, H. (2007) Sexual Boundary Violations by Health Professionals – An Overview of the Published Empirical Literature. London: CHRE.

Subotsky, F. (2010) Abuse of the Doctor-Patient Relationship. London: RCPsych Publications.

Totton, N. (2001). 'Scapegoats and Sacred Cows: Towards Good Enough Conflict Resolution.' In R. Casemore (ed.) *Surviving Complaints against Counsellors and Psychotherapists: Towards Understanding and Healing*. London: PCCS.

Part II

SHOT BY BOTH SIDES

THE THERAPEUTIC MILIEU UNDER ATTACK

Cannon to right of them,
Cannon to left of them,
Cannon in front of them
Volley'd and thunder'd…

From *The Charge of the Light Brigade*,
Alfred Lord Tennyson (1855)

Chapter 6

'MIRROR MIRROR'
Parallel Processes in Forensic Institutions

Gwen Adshead

In this chapter Gwen Adshead opens the second part of the book in considering the implications of long periods of treatment, occasionally involving a lifetime of confinement. She examines the ways in which forensic settings reflect the problematic dynamics of the families of origin of their patients. She argues that the 'fire' of this book's title generates 'an emotional heat' fuelled by the interaction of the patient and staff groupings and their respective patterns of attachment. She highlights the fact that many patients have insecure attachments, showing a range of abnormal behaviours when distressed, but she also cites evidence that some insecurely attached children grow up to be 'compulsive caregivers' in adulthood, choosing professional caring as a career. These dynamics are reflected in a process of malignant mirroring between staff and patients and across the different layers of the organisation. She suggests that awareness of these multiple reflections helps maintain integrity of therapeutic purpose.

INTRODUCTION

Long-stay residential care was the mainstay of psychiatric treatment across Europe and the USA until it was replaced by community programmes in the late 20th century. Almost the only services now that offer long-stay (two or more years) residential care are forensic psychiatric services that admit people whose disorders and behaviours have frightened others. Patients admitted to these services often spend five or more years in hospital; and those whose behaviour appears particularly risky, whose offences are inexplicable or whose disorders are resistant to treatment, may stay much longer (Dell and Robertson 1988).

It is sadly no secret that abuses and lapses of professional care take place in such settings; and they are often stigmatised and stigmatising institutions to live and work in. In this chapter, I will explore how complex (and at times toxic) group dynamics may help to explain why it is sometimes hard for staff to think in forensic settings. I will draw on psychoanalytic, group analytic and attachment theory; and argue that the 'fire' under which staff have to think is a complex emotional heat that is generated by an interaction of group dynamics and toxic attachments in both patient and professional groups. I will close by offering some 'golden rules' for staff groups.

MIRRORING IN GROUPS

We are social animals whose primate heritage requires us to live in groups. To do this successfully, we need a 'social mind': one that has the capacity to appreciate that others have thoughts, intentions and experience (Dunbar 2003). This mentalising capacity has a number of sub-capacities and faculties, including the capacity to 'read' other people's emotions and respond to them. In non-human primates this process is not conscious, symbolised or reflected on; but in human primates, the expanded neo-cortex makes self-experience and language possible, which in turn makes group living more successful (Dunbar 1993).

Early group analytic theorists (e.g. Foulkes 1964; Pines 1998) noted that group members would seem to 'mirror' the emotions and communications of other group members; or unconsciously act out the behaviour and communication of key figures discussed in group members' narratives. Such a process could be positive and support the formation of rich interpersonal relating; but it could also be toxic or 'malignant' (Zinkin 1983) and interfere with group process and development.

We now know that this 'mirroring' process in groups is the social manifestation of that 'social mind' described in primates, and it is a form of empathic non-verbal communication mediated through specific 'mirror' neurons in the brain. Mirror neurons are activated (at least in monkeys) by imitative interaction. In humans, mirroring may be understood as the persistence of a form of non-verbal and unconscious communication, which can be elaborated and extended by more conscious aspects of the self-reflective system, including the faculties of empathy and sympathy (which are mediated by a separate neural network in the frontal neo-cortex).

Such a rich array of emotional communication is vital for the making and maintaining of social relationships in groups, which underpins group survival. However, primate life is not always easy or pleasant; and hostility, rage, disgust and shame are primary emotions that are a natural part of the social life of primates (De Waal 2001; Sapolsky 2002). Negative emotions will inevitably be communicated within and between groups; especially those emotions that involve the gaze and response of others, such as shame and disgust. Groups typically reject members who shame and disgust them, or demean them in terms of rank: this process is highly stressful and reduces life expectancy and well-being (Sapolsky 2005).

Any group of people living together for any length of time will therefore be emotionally affected by one another through processes of 'emotional contagion', one of which is the mirroring process, which is non-conscious, non-verbal and inevitable. Such mirroring processes are a challenge to traditional models of professionalism in health care, which usually state either 1) that good professionals don't have feelings about patients, or 2) that if they do, they should only be positive feelings, characterised as a kind of detached sympathy.

However, this traditional professional ideal does not represent best practice, but rather a Victorian ideal of masculinity (Micale 2008). Health care professionals cannot help but have feelings about their patients, both conscious and unconscious; and I now turn to attachment theory as an explanatory paradigm for understanding those feelings.

REPRESENTATIONS OF ATTACHMENTS IN MIND: INDIVIDUAL AND GROUP

Attachment theory integrates psychoanalysis with the ethological study of social animals; and starts from the position that man is essentially a social animal who needs relationships for survival, and whose early relationships with carers have unique characteristics that influence the development of later relationships (Bowlby 1980; Holmes 1993). Attachment behaviour is any form of behaviour which results in a person attaining or maintaining proximity to an 'attachment figure', an identified individual who is experienced as stronger or less vulnerable at that moment (Weiss 1991). Such behaviour is most obvious when people are frightened, fatigued or sick, and is assuaged by comforting and caregiving (George and Solomon 1996). It can be seen throughout the life cycle, especially in emergencies, and its biological function appears to be the protection of the developing and vulnerable organism. The formation of attachment bonds results in neurochemical and neurocytological changes in the brain, especially in the prefrontal cortex that regulates conscious and unconscious feeling (see Kraemer 1992; Schore 1994 for review).

To say of a person that he is attached to, or has an attachment to another, is to say that he is strongly disposed to seek proximity to and contact with that individual, and to do so especially when distressed, anxious, injured or vulnerable. Bowlby suggested that the nature and quality of the attachment is represented in the mind as an unconscious 'internal working model' of both how to seek care and how to give it. The attachment system in mind is therefore a mental representation (with both conscious and unconscious elements) of a dynamic system that involves a care-giver and a care-elicitor (George and Solomon 1996). Attachment representations work as a kind of internal homeostatic mechanism for modulating anxiety, fear and distress.

When the attachment system is stimulated (i.e. when the individual is in need, pain or danger), it produces neural signals that in turn stimulate physiological effects that influence thought and feeling in the neo-cortex. In a feedback loop, these thoughts and feelings produce more physiological manifestations of anxiety and arousal, which agitate the attachment system further. A 'secure' system makes it possible to process anxiety and arousal effectively, which includes being able to reach out to carers and be comfortable with vulnerability. An 'insecure' system can process neither anxiety nor arousal well enough at times of distress, and those with insecure attachment representations will struggle to form useful relationships with care providers (Henderson 1974).

These attachment representations include representations of *groups*, of which one is a member. It is known that babies as young as seven months are aware of a distinction between family members and those who are outside the family. This suggests that they have already formed a conceptual representation of the differences that signify 'my group of people' and 'not my group of people'. Josselson (1995) has suggested that normal psychological development includes a group representation which expands as new people are added to the 'group-in-mind'. This representation of 'groupishness' (Miller 1998; see also Chapter 14) is arguably part of the attachment system; and will affect how an individual relates to groups in the future, both work and therapeutic (Glenn 1987; Marrone 1998). Group attachment systems may be secure or insecure in the same way as individual attachment systems; and may account for why some people find it easier to make therapeutic use of groups, while others seem to make toxic attachments to groups.

ATTACHMENT REPRESENTATIONS IN CLINICAL SETTINGS

Theoretically, we might expect to find high levels of insecure attachment in psychiatric services users, which may make it difficult for those service-users to relate effectively to professional carers. Research into attachment representations in clinical and non-clinical populations (Bakermans-Kranenburg and van IJzendoorn 2009) provides supportive evidence for these hypotheses. As predicted, the majority of people in *non-clinical groups* (58%) describe 'secure' attachment relationships: they seek care effectively when distressed, are 'comfortable' with the experience of being distressed (insofar as they do not experience high levels of fear) and anticipate positive outcomes with carers.

However, in *clinical* groups, less than 20 per cent of people are rated as securely attached, implying that most psychiatric care seekers have insecure attachment representations in their minds. There is also evidence that insecure people show a range of abnormal behaviours when they are distressed. They tend to either freeze, panic or deny feelings of distress, or they oscillate around seeking care and then withdrawing from it (Hesse 2008; van IJzendoorn and Bakermans-Kranenburg 2003). Specifically, insecure subjects struggle to regulate the proximity inherent in caring attachment relationships because their internal working models are not able to do the necessary psychological work of regulating affects of anxiety, distress and anger. There is a particular sub-group of insecure individuals who describe highly disorganised attachment representations and behaviours (usually after maltreatment in childhood), and unresolved distress from trauma and loss experiences. Disorganised attachment in children is characterised by confused and inconsistent attachment behaviour (van IJzendoorn and Bakermans-Kranenburg 2003) and is associated with the development of clinical symptoms in adolescence such as dissociative phenomena and psychotic thinking. Disorganised attachment representations are much more frequently found in clinical groups (20%) than non-clinical (6%), and theoretically at least are likely to have disorganised relationships with carers when distressed.

Lastly, there is evidence that insecure attachment representations in the mind have a negative impact on care-giving behaviour in adulthood (van IJzendoorn 1995). Bowlby postulated that some insecurely attached children would grow up to be 'compulsive caregivers' in adulthood (Bowlby 1960), which may be relevant to those who choose professional caring as a career. Insecure attachment in adults is associated with atypical care-giving behaviours with infants and older children (Goldberg *et al.* 2003) and parents who abuse or neglect their children are far more likely to be categorised as insecure than secure in attachment terms (Adshead and Bluglass 2005).

The implications of this research for forensic residential services are significant. If psychiatric services users generally have high levels of insecure attachment, then we may anticipate that the majority of forensic patients will have insecure attachment patterns, which means that they may find it hard to make and maintain therapeutic relationships with professional carers (Norton 1996; Dozier *et al.* 2001). We know that 80 per cent of forensic populations have experienced significant maltreatment in childhood, so they are likely to have developed disorganised attachment systems, and have unresolved trauma and loss experiences (Adshead 2004), which means that this forensic group may relate to professional carers in particularly bizarre and dysfunctional ways, including aggression, fear or toxic enmeshment.

This research also implies that there may a sub-group of staff with insecure attachment histories, who may be at risk of showing atypical or dysfunctional care behaviours or may be more likely to get caught up in toxic attachment relationships with equally insecure patients. Some staff may have become care-givers because of their own insecure childhoods, and although this could be turned to good use in some circumstances, it is possible that this group may be vulnerable to lapses of professional care, such as professional boundary violations.

Lastly, we may anticipate that those with highly insecure and disorganised attachment systems may struggle to attach to therapeutic groups, or relate trustfully to them. The paradox here is that recovery of a more pro-social identity entails attachment to groups of some sort, not least because social isolation is a significant risk factor for violence.

THE EFFECTS OF UNCONSCIOUS ANXIETY IN PROFESSIONAL CARERS

In 1959, Menzies Lyth published a ground-breaking study of why professional carers (in this case, nurses on general medical wards) were leaving the profession midway through training or taking excessive sick leave. She concluded that the nursing staff were 'unconsciously distressed' by many aspects of the nursing process, such as performing intimate and distasteful tasks which can arouse feelings of disgust, fear, hatred or even excitement. Nurses might be also unconsciously envious of the care their patients received or aggrieved when patients did not improve or appear grateful for their care.

Menzies Lyth suggested that collectively the nursing staff developed social defences to enable them to cope with the intolerable feelings aroused by working in difficult and stressful environments. These defences were unconscious and helped to keep the anxiety unconscious also. They chiefly took the form of behaviours that helped the nurses avoid being in personal contact with patients, such as referring to the patients by their diagnoses or symptoms, or allocating so many patients to one nurse that they could not possibly be seen in a shift. Defences could also take the form of ritualistic tasks, such as checking and re-checking every action or decision. Lastly, there was an emphasis at senior levels on the development of emotional detachment as a sign of 'good' professional behaviour. A feature of a 'good nurse' was that they were willing to move from ward to ward with no notice, leaving distressed patients behind without a thought; and no suggestion that either patients or staff might have feelings about this.

Nurses were found to minimise their anxiety by the use of immature defences such as denial, splitting and projection (Menzies Lyth 1959). These immature defences are commonly used by everyone at times of stress but, in the work situation, staff projected unwanted feelings that they could not bear to feel into other members of the nursing team. For example, teams became split into those nurses who were 'responsible' and those who were seen as 'irresponsible'. The 'responsible' nurses complained that the 'irresponsible' ones needed to be constantly supervised and disciplined, which led to more and more ritualistic checking behaviour, and prevented the 'irresponsible' staff from actually learning to do their jobs in a responsible way. Projection was not confined to fellow staff; anger and frustration of the work was also projected into patients, who were seen as endlessly demanding and troublesome.

Menzies Lyth concluded that these social defences operated to help the individual and the institution avoid the conscious experience of anxiety, guilt and uncertainty. But she also pointed out that such immature defences failed to do the job intended; not only did they not relieve anxiety but further anxiety was in fact generated by the defence itself, and conscious reactions to it. Staff still felt anxious and distressed, but the social defences meant that they were not allowed to know their feelings or express them. No attempt was made to enable the individual nurses to confront and face their anxieties and distress. They were therefore unable to develop a capacity to bear these anxieties more effectively. Without a capacity to manage their distress, it was inevitable that staff would drop out of training or go sick, leading to the staffing problems that were the 'presenting problem'.

Menzies Lyth's work has been applied widely, including in general mental health and forensic settings (Hinshelwood and Skogstad 2000; Lowdell and Adshead 2009). It is important work, for two reasons: first, because it shows how individual defences can become mirrored and intensified in group situations in institutions, ultimately becoming mirrored and enacted in institutional policy and procedures. Second, it demonstrates how the care of the sick is stressful and distressing, and how impossible it is for staff *not* to have negative feelings about their patients from time to time. From an attachment theory perspective also, I would argue that residential care in hospital maximally activates care-eliciting and caregiving systems in both staff and patients; it is also possible that some of the staff in Menzies Lyth's study were particularly vulnerable to using psychotic defences because of their own attachment histories.

THE PSYCHOLOGICAL DEMANDS OF RESIDENTIAL FORENSIC CARE

An important feature of forensic secure care is that it entails long-term residential care where patients are not just receiving treatment, they are also living their lives. This type of care, which used to be the main form of psychiatric treatment, is now almost exclusively found in secure settings. Long-stay residential care makes specific demands on staff, as described by Miller and Gwynne (1972) in their study of residential institutions for the physically handicapped and chronically sick – a group who used to be called 'the incurables'.

Using Menzies Lyth's approach, Miller and Gwynne found that long stay (even life-time) residential institutions tended to operate either a 'warehousing' or 'horticultural' model of care. In the 'warehousing' model, patients were classified by diagnosis, and treated as utterly dependent objects, rather than people with lives to lead. The horticultural model emphasised growth of capabilities and independence, but sometimes overlooked patients' real need to be cared for. What Miller and Gywnne noted was the residents' experience of rejection, isolation from their communities and 'social death' because of the damage caused by their physical disability. They also noted the lack of a social discourse for thinking or talking about those situations where adults are dependent on other adults for long periods.

These studies of psychodynamics in health care institutions have disturbing implications for forensic residential care. If toxic anxiety and institutional acting out are generated in general medical care (where there is an average stay of six weeks), how much more anxiety and distress may be generated in care of patients that goes on for years? Menzies Lyth describes general medical nurses struggling with feelings of disgust when dealing with patients' bodies, but in forensic settings staff may have to struggle with feeling disgust and fear in response to what their patients have done with their bodies and to other bodies, and the disgusting or horrifying things that may be going on in patients' minds. Note that fear and disgust may be conscious reactions but staff may also struggle to be conscious of less socially acceptable feelings, such as hatred, revenge or vicarious excitement.

Forensic secure care has much in common with homes for the 'incurables', not least because there is a strong public (and perhaps professional) perception that offender patients are beyond help (see also Chapter 3). Forensic patients are rejected, isolated and experience 'social death': they have arguably acquired a distorted identity that they will not be allowed to shake off, no matter how much they try (Williams *et al.* 2011). Forensic patients are 'disabled' not only by their psychopathology but also by the perception of their dangerousness, which frightens others, and justifies the removal of autonomy and independence.

Miller and Gwynne describe how the inner lives of the residents are expressed in the caring relationship and the effect this can have on staff behaviour (p.137). If this is true, then we may expect some disturbed and disturbing behaviour in forensic settings, not just by individual staff members (see Chapter 5) but also in terms of institutional policy and practice (see Chapter 4), as has sadly been demonstrated by the repeated public inquiries into forensic residential care (Davies 2004; see also Box 6.1). In the first Ashworth Inquiry, there was evidence that staff had been physically abusive to patients. In the second Ashworth Inquiry, it became clear that staff had either colluded with patients in rule-breaking behaviour, or turned a blind eye to it, or not noticed it.

BOX 6.1 EVIDENCE THAT THE PRIMARY TASK GOES WRONG IN FORENSIC SETTINGS

- *Abusive care.* Rampton, the first Ashworth Inquiry (Blom Cooper 1992).

- *Collusive care.* The second Ashworth Inquiry (Fallon 1999); press accounts of sexual boundary violations by staff at Broadmoor hospital.

- *Neglectful care.* Patient deaths in Broadmoor hospital: one homicide (NCAS London 2009) and multiple suicides.

These might seem like different kinds of problem, but in reality they are not. They are sad examples of how staff can get caught up in the emotions that forensic patients unconsciously evoke in them. Staff may have conscious reactions to the patients (which may be difficult enough to manage), such as hostility, rage, contempt and fear. They will almost certainly have *unconscious* reactions to the patients, when the relationship triggers off reminders of past relationships: either the patient's past or the staff member's past.

In Ashworth One, we can guess that the staff must have perceived the patients as especially provocative and threatening, to have reached the point where they used violence against patients (as opposed to organised restraint or some other socially sanctioned response). It may be that there was something about the presentation of the patients that triggered unconsciously in staff fears about their own capacity to become disorganised and anxiety about their capacity to contain the patients. Many forensic patients (especially with personality disorder) are anxious about containment of feelings, and they look to others to ensure they will not be overwhelmed. This anxiety is then mirrored by the staff, who may act violently in response to their own sense of panic that they are not in control. If in reality staff numbers are down, or the ward is particularly stressed, then the chance of staff feeling helpless and panicky is increased, which in turn may increase the risk of them acting in a hostile way to patients. None of the above is an excuse for unprofessional behaviour, but it does provide a framework for understanding what happened and how it might be prevented.

Similarly, with Ashworth Two, it is possible that the staff felt equally overwhelmed and made helpless by the patients' cruelty and hopelessness. It is possible that they failed to notice what was going on and/or failed to take action because they felt there was no point in noticing or acting. In this way, they may have unconsciously identified with the victims of their patients, and also the victim part of each patient's history. Victims of violence characteristically 'freeze' and become passive in the face of danger; they can also experience overwhelming hopelessness and helplessness, which further increases passivity.

Staff may also have made an identification with the cruel and delinquent part of each patient's mind. Both cruelty and successful rule-breaking can lead to a (usually brief) sense of triumph that may have contributed to a cheerful atmosphere on the ward, which both staff and patients enjoyed. It is very human not to want to disturb what appears to be working well, especially when this means taking on people who have been violent and cruel in the past. Rule-breaking patients who wanted to deceive staff may have gone out of their way to be pleasant and engaging, in a way which is hard to resist in secure settings, which are often otherwise so turbulent. The sad truth is also that staff members may be more trusting than the patients, which can lead to collusion.

Colluding with rule-breaking may also be more likely in staff who themselves had a history of rule-breaking in their own childhoods, or who had also had experiences of being abused. Given the prevalence of childhood abuse and neglect in the general population, it would be surprising if some survivors did not become health care professionals; indeed, there is some reason to think that one way to cope with having had an insecure childhood is to become a professional carer in adulthood (Bowlby 1960).

It seems difficult for large social structures, like organised work groups, to learn from disasters and we can only surmise that institutions that are traumatised by their own failures suffer from complex trauma reactions that include dissociation and blanks where memories should be (Hopper 2012). People may be speechless after a disaster for many years; articulating what went wrong could be painful and shameful. It is understandably easier then for forensic institutions to identify a scapegoat, expel them from the group and then carry on as before; a parallel and mirror of how the forensic patients were admitted to the forensic institution in the first place.

INTENSIFICATION OF MIRRORING IN MULTIPLE GROUPS

To understand boundary violations in forensic health care, we must appreciate the intensification of mirror phenomena because of the presence of different types of human group (Figure 6.1). The patient group on a ward acts like a toxic family group, where there are multiple toxic attachments to professional carers and to peers. Wards can resemble the mind of a patient, which may be superficially calm and composed, but underneath there is real incoherence, madness and danger. Each patient brings not only his or her capacity for cruelty and causing fear in others; they also bring their histories of fear, helplessness and hopelessness. Staff must provide a type of intimacy in which awful things can be spoken of: either terrible feelings in the here-and-now, or the reliving of horrific events from the past. They must be emotionally available for patients, but at the same time be aware that some patients struggle with continuing wishes to harm, deceive or corrupt others. Perhaps what is most important is that the nurse understands that their own emotional response to their work may be a function of what the patient is evoking in his or herself.

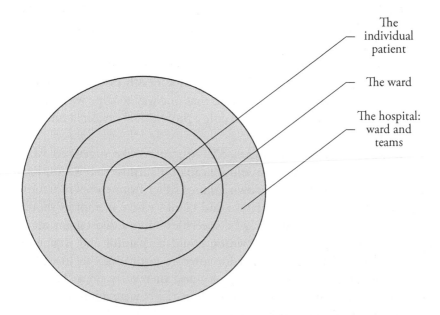

Figure 6.1 An ecological model of a secure hospital: made up of concentric groups of people carrying out different tasks for the group in the centre who are the group of patients

Staff on a forensic ward themselves form a group of people who have to relate to each other and rely on each other in settings that are both stressful and dull. This combination of boredom that alternates unpredictably with high anxiety has been reported as being particularly stressful in occupational terms. Staff in secure settings must not only attend to the patients' needs; they must also attend to the organisation's need for policies and procedures to be met to an ever more demanding standard. Some of these are essential for security and risk management (and therefore generate an urgency and anxiety) while some seem irrelevant, futile and facile; often because they relate to quality-of-care indicators that were devised for other non-psychiatric or non-forensic settings. The same tasks may be repeatedly requested by different managerial groups at different times, reflecting the huge managerial anxiety present in forensic institutions (Armstrong 2005, p.46).

All these tasks reduce the time staff have to spend with patients, just as Menzies Lyth described. However, although this may be consciously (and unconsciously) welcomed by staff who want to get away from patients, reduced time with patients increases both the risk that some aspect of danger will be missed, and anxiety about that risk, which then stimulates more and more behaviours designed to reduce risk and reduce contact with the patient who is the source of the risk (see below).

Case example

Bill kills a family member and is admitted to a medium secure unit. After admission, he is antagonistic to staff, disparaging of therapy and physically aggressive. Eventually he is transferred to a high secure hospital because of his violence to staff. Other family members give him the message that he will soon be released and live a normal life with them. Bill is generally disparaging of all types of therapy, except for individual therapy with a young woman with whom he flirts. He barely engages with ward and offence-based group therapies.

In the high secure hospital, staff give him parole that would normally be given to patients who have completed therapy and are not antagonistic to staff. Against the advice of his therapists, Bill is transferred from the high secure hospital to another medium secure facility. Bill is initially compliant then becomes more aggressive and intimidating to staff. Eventually he is returned to the high secure hospital, in an event which is *an exact repetition* of the violence that led to his earlier admission. As Bill is escorted away by the police, he can be heard shouting, 'You can't do this to me, I'm not a patient.'

All work groups struggle with task completion, and if the task is complex then completion may be difficult. Groups go off task in a variety of ways: fight, flight, pairing, or adopting a rigid dominance hierarchy in which those at the bottom are ridiculed and belittled, and those at the top ignore information that might prevent disasters (Armstrong 2005; Surowiecki 2004). Such hierarchies also encourage internal competition between individuals and sub-groups of workers, which causes friction, resentment and inevitably failure to complete the task at hand.

TAKING CARE: RELATIONAL SECURITY AND PSYCHOLOGICAL MINDEDNESS IN FORENSIC INSTITUTIONS

So how might forensic services respond creatively to the challenge of working with highly disturbed people and help both staff and systems to function better? First, some acceptance of the difficulty and complexity of the task is essential. Improved awareness, acceptance and understanding will not abolish the problems but may offer more functional ways of coping with anxiety and distress.

Bowlby (1988) hoped that his attachment paradigm would make it easier to understand toxic therapeutic relationships as places where patients inevitably re-enact insecure attachment behaviours with carers. But if the therapeutic relationship could offer a new 'secure base' to enable patients to manage their attachments better, then this would offer the possibility of more 'secure' ways of managing care seeking and giving with others in the future. This concept of a 'secure' therapeutic base has particular resonance when applied to forensic settings (Adshead 2004). Forensic patients need to become more *psychologically* secure and the physical security system imposes space and time to think and develop psychological security. Inevitably, patients will enact their attachment anxieties in the here-and-now of residential life: not only in therapy, but generally with professional carers and patients on the ward. Each ward functions as a group of people living and working together in ways that affect one another: the staff and patients on a single ward together make up a large group (about 50 people) who function like a mini-institution, or a large extended family. These large groups need help if they are not to become gangs, or battlefields. Help includes reflective spaces for staff and patients: spaces which look directly at relational processes within and between different sub-groups of people (Hartley and Kennard 2009; see also Chapter 14).

Staff need to be psychologically secure enough to manage the conscious anxiety their job entails. They also need to be given room to become more aware of their unconscious anxieties. If this does not happen, then the anxiety is likely to be acted out in atypical and odd behaviours at work – a mirror of the ways that insecure patients act out their anxiety in bizarre and risky behaviours. Typically staff enact their anxiety in forensic settings by breaking the rules, most commonly in minor ways by being inconsistent with patients and each other, but (rarely) in more major ways by physical boundary breaches and/or turning a blind eye to such behaviour (Davies 2004; Adshead 2012).

The awareness, acceptance and understanding process needs to be taken up by all workers in forensic settings, not just nurses on the wards. The ward staff are first 'in the line of fire'; but like the infantry in battle, they are connected to and managed by senior practitioners and managers of the services who are responsible for what happens on the wards as much as the front-line staff. There is good evidence that non-ward staff (such as doctors or senior service health care managers) are just as vulnerable to acting out and boundary breaches as anyone else (Main 1977). Psychiatrists are particularly at risk of being formally investigated for failures in team work (NCAS 2009), which suggests either that psychiatry attracts insecure individuals who relate poorly in groups or that mental health teams are groups that struggle with terrible anxiety, and those who lead them may easily be scapegoated (Sarkar 2009).

We also need to take better care of ourselves, and understand that this is a major aspect of keeping the boundary between our professional and personal identities (see Chapter 15). The literature on boundary-breaking professionals indicates that they are often facing an attachment crisis in their personal lives, such as the birth of a child, bereavement or family distress. If their personal attachment systems are activated, but no care is available at home, then these professionals may come to work hoping that the workplace will soothe them or take care of their distress, especially if they are coming to a hospital! If this does not occur, then they may respond with angry outbursts and behavioural displays of distress; or they may seek support from patients, or be gratified by patients' attachment to them in ways that are risky, and enhance the risk of sexual boundary violations. In forensic settings, this is especially risky because some patients are predatory and become excited by others' vulnerability, and may be only too keen to engage in breaches of security.

So supervision and line management need to be flexible and skilled enough to make it possible to talk about personal matters, and need to engage with the reality that personal attachments may affect professional performance. This means that supervisors and managers need to become skilled in the types of conversation that need to take place and it is no longer acceptable for 'supervision' of a health care professional to focus only on management targets or professional goals. The expectation works both ways: supervisees will be expected to reflect on their own psychological health and well-being and be prepared to explore the boundary between personal and the professional identities, and the tension or relationship between these two identities. The supervisory skill then lies in exploring just enough of the personal to understand the professional issue and keeping the boundaries between supervision, management, friendship and therapy.

CONCLUSION: GOLDEN RULES FOR RELATIONAL SECURITY IN FORENSIC SYSTEMS

Note that these conclusions apply to both staff and patients.

- No one is allowed to rubbish anyone else. Constructive criticism or comment is fine, but not disparagement or denigration.

- If you hurt someone's feelings, apologise. This doesn't mean accepting error or fault; only regret that someone important to the system felt hurt.

- People can, and must, be allowed to be appropriately angry and distressed about events or changes that affect them without being attacked for it.

- Build up pro-social banking in good times, that is praising good work, and thanking people for doing extra or contributing to someone else's work.

- Promote curiosity: the culture of enquiry. The ability of group members to ask questions is usually the sign of a healthy group process.

- Triumph and disaster are imposters: they may not tell the truth about a person or an institution.

REFERENCES

Adshead, G. (2004) 'Three Degrees of Security: Attachment and Forensic Institutions.' In F. Pfäfflin and G. Adshead (eds) *A Matter of Security: The Application of Attachment Theory to Forensic Psychiatry and Psychotherapy.* London: Jessica Kingsley Publishers.

Adshead, G. (2012) 'What the eye doesn't see: relationships, boundaries and forensic mental health.' In A. Aiyegbusi and G. Kelly (eds) *Professional and Therapeutic Boundaries in Forensic Mental Health Practice.* London: Jessica Kingsley Publishers.

Adshead, G. and Bluglass, K. (2005) 'Attachment representations in FIP mothers.' *British Journal of Psychiatry* 187, 328–333.

Armstrong, D. (2005) *The Organisation in the Mind.* London: Karnac.

Bakermans-Kranenburg, M. and van IJzendoorn, M. (2009) 'The first 10,000 Adult Attachment interviews: distribution of adult attachment representations in clinical and non-clinical groups.' *Attachment and Human Development 11*, 3, 223–263.

Blom Cooper, L. (1992) *Report of the Committee of Inquiry into Complaints about Ashworth Hospital.* London: Stationery Office CM 2028.

Bowlby, J. (1960) *Attachment and Loss, Vol.1. Attachment.* London: Hogarth Press.

Bowlby, J. (1980) *Attachment and Loss, Vol.3. Loss.* London: Hogarth Press. Pimlico edition 1998.

Bowlby, J. (1988) *A Secure Base.* London: Routledge.

Davies, S. (2004) 'Toxic Institutions.' In P. Campling, S. Davies and G. Farquharson (eds) *From Toxic Institutions to Therapeutic Environments.* London: Gaskell.

Dell, S. and Robertson, G. (1988) *Sentenced to Hospital: Offenders in Broadmoor.* Maudsley Monograph. Oxford: OUP.

De Waal, F. (2001) *The Ape and the Sushi Master: Cultural Reflections of a Primatologist.* New York: Basic Books.

Dozier, M., Lomax, L., Tyrrell, C. and Lee, S. (2001) 'The challenge of treatment for clients with a dismissing state of mind.' *Attachment & Human Behaviour 3*, 1, 62–76.

Dunbar, R. (1993) 'Co-evolution of neocortical size, group size and language in humans.' *Brain and Behavioural Sciences 16*, 681–735.

Dunbar R. (2003) 'The social brain: mind, language and society in evolutionary perspective.' *Annual Review Anthropology 32*, 163–181.

Fallon Report (1999) *Report of the Committee of Inquiry into the Personality Disorder Unit at Ashworth Hospital.* London: Stationery Office.

Foulkes, S. (1964) *Therapeutic Group Analysis.* London: Maresfield.

George, C. and Solomon, J. (1996) 'Representational models of relationships: links between care giving and attachment.' *Infant Mental Health Journal 17*, 198–216.

Glenn, L. (1987) 'Attachment theory and group analysis: the group matrix as a secure base.' *Group Analysis 20*, 2, 109–117.

Goldberg, S., Benoit, D., Blokland, K. and Madigan, S. (2003) 'Atypical maternal behaviour, maternal representation and infant disorganized attachment.' *Development and Psychopathology 15*, 239–257.

Hartley, P. and Kennard, D. (2009) *Staff Support Groups in the Helping Professions.* London: Routledge.

Henderson, S. (1974) 'Care eliciting behaviour in man.' *Journal of Nervous and Mental Disease 159*, 172–181.

Hesse, E. (2008) 'The Adult Attachment Interview.' In J. Cassidy and P. Shaver (eds) *Handbook of Attachment* (2nd edition). New York: Guilford.

Hinshelwood, R. and Skogstad, W. (2000) *Observing Organisations: Anxiety, Defence and Culture in Health Care.* London: Routledge.

Holmes, J. (1993) *John Bowlby and Attachment Theory.* London: Routledge.

Hopper, E. (2012) *Trauma in Organisations.* London: Karnac.

Josselson, R.-E. (1995) *The Space between us: Exploring the Dimensions of Human Relationships.* London: Sage.

Kraemer, G. (1992) 'A psychobiological theory of attachment.' *Behavioural and Brain Sciences 15*, 493–541.

Lowdell, A. and Adshead, G. (2009) 'The Best Defence: Institutional Defences Against Anxiety in Forensic Services.' In A. Aiyegbusi and J. Clarke-Moore (eds) *Therapeutic Relationships with Offenders: An Introduction to the Psychodynamics of Forensic Mental Health Nursing.* London: Jessica Kingsley Publishers.

Main, T. (1977) 'Traditional psychiatric defences against close encounters with patients.' *Canadian Psychiatric Association 22*, 457–466.

Marrone, M. (1998) *Attachment and Interaction.* London: Jessica Kingsley Publishers.

Menzies Lyth, I. (1959) 'The Functioning of Social Systems as Defence Against Anxiety: A Report on a Study of the Nursing Service of a General Hospital.' In *Containing Anxiety in Institutions. Volume 1.* London: Free Association Books.

Micale, M. (2008) *Hysterical Men: The Hidden History of Male Nervous Illness.* Harvard: Harvard University Press.

Miller, E. (1998) 'A note on protomental systems and "groupishness": Bion's Basic assumptions revisited.' *Human Relations 5*, 12, 1495–1508.

Miller, E. and Gwynne, G. (1972) *A Life Apart: A Pilot Study of Residential Institutions for the Physically Handicapped and the Young Chronic Sick.* London: Tavistock Publications.

NCAS (2009) *National Clinical Assessment Service: The First Eight Years.* London: NCAS.

Norton, K. (1996) 'Management of difficult personality disorder patients.' *Advances in Psychiatric Treatment 2*, 202–210.

Pines, M. (1998) 'Reflections on Mirroring.' In M. Pines (ed) *Circular Reflections: Selected Papers on Group Analysis and Psychoanalysis.* London: Jessica Kingsley Publishers.

Sapolsky, R. (2002) *A Primate's Memoir: My Unconventional Life Among the Baboons*. New York: Simon & Schuster.

Sapolsky, R. (2005) 'The influence of social hierarchies on primate health.' *Science 308*, 648–652.

Sarkar, S. (2009) 'The dance of dissent: managing conflict in health care organisations.' *Psychoanalytic Psychotherapy 23*, 2, 121–135.

Schore, A. (1994) *Affect Regulation and the Origin of the Self: The Neurobiology of Emotional Development*. New Jersey: Laurence Erlbaum.

Surowiecki, J. (2004) *The Wisdom of Crowds: Why the Many are Smarter Than the Few*. London: Doubleday. Abacus 2005.

Van IJzendoorn, M. (1995) 'Adult attachment representations, parental responsiveness and infant attachment: a meta-analysis on the predictive validity of the Adult Attachment Interview.' *Psychological Bulletin 117*, 3, 387–403.

van IJzendoorn, M. and Bakermans-Kranenburg, M. (2003) 'Attachment disorders and disorganised attachment: similar and different.' *Attachment and Human Development 5*, 3, 313–320.

Weiss, R. (1991) 'The Attachment Bond in Childhood and Adulthood.' In C. Parkes, J. Stevenson Hinde and P. Marris (eds) *Attachment across the Life Cycle*. London: Routledge.

Williams, A., Moore, E., Adshead, G., McDowell, A. and Tapp, J. (2011) 'Including the excluded: high secure user perspectives on stigma, discrimination and recovery.' *British Journal of Forensic Practice*.

Zinkin, L. (1983) 'Malignant mirroring.' *Group Analysis 16*, 2, 113–126.

Chapter 7

SINGLE-SEX UNITS AS A DEFENCE AGAINST ANXIETY?

Anna Motz

In this chapter Anna Motz discusses the particular case of the mixed gender therapeutic milieu, which has come under intense cross-fire in recent years. She explores whether the trend towards single-sex wards offers or denies the women a milieu in which they are able to process their traumatic experiences. Motz continues the themes both of destructive motherhood which was introduced in Neeld and Clarke's chapter and of the mirroring of family dynamics explored by Adshead, in presenting the case of Lily, the subject of abusive mothering and a perpetrator of child abduction. Through this case material she investigates the unconscious basis for single-sex units and their potential to re-awaken primitive fears of sexuality, leading to the exile and punishment of these women.

INTRODUCTION

Over recent years in the UK there has been a governmental drive to establish women-only units within mental health services. Mainstreaming Women's Mental Health (Department of Health 2002) has become established. This is the separate provision of male and female treatment facilities and the creation of environments that cater to the specific needs of women, protecting them from exposure to the very situations that initially traumatised them, for instance proximity to sexually predatory men.

The concern that women with long histories of physical, emotional and sexual abuse will be harmed by close contact with aggressive antisocial men is well founded. I have directly witnessed how trauma repeated itself, how vulnerable women with little sense of their own worth would hide away in frightening mixed environments, or form relationships with men who betrayed and violated them, recapitulating their early trauma (Motz 2008).

But in identifying dangerous relationships with men and reducing the risk of their repetition as our central task, are we not ignoring the fact that in these enclosed, intense settings, destructive relationships between women may also get repeated, and magnified? Is it possible to use principles of relational security and attachment models to rectify the damage of these early relationships, or will the disturbance of these women, and their fears of care, lead to traumatic re-enactments even within single-sex units?

While the exclusive provision of women-only units addresses the profound differences in male and female presentations of disturbance, violence and mental illness, it is also possible to see it as a defensive manoeuvre; it may ignore the complexity and potential destructiveness of women-to-women relationships and, sometimes falsely identifies the male as so different, and so toxic, that he must be exiled to another setting altogether (for other material on the projection of other-ness and the dynamics of difference see Chapters 2 and 12).

Despite its rational basis, and sound principles of protective care, it is possible that this project is actually a search for an idealised 'mother ward'. Such a quest may not only lead to disappointment, but carries the risk of re-creating a fused and toxic symbolic coupling of mother and child, in which the helpful presence of a third term, a male, is absent.

At the same time it is undeniable that women have radically different histories and trajectories into secure services than men do, and some would be harmed if placed in locked wards with predatory males from whom they couldn't escape (Bland, Mezey and Dolan 1999; Coid *et al.* 2003). Some of these women, but not all, are so vulnerable to being abused that they would be placed in active danger if they shared a ward with men, where they could be drawn into exploitative and damaging relationships.

In this chapter I raise the question of whether this drive for exclusively single-sex units within medium and high secure mental health settings is actually regressive or progressive.

CLINICAL ILLUSTRATION:
A WOMAN WHO TOOK A BABY

Lily was a 50-year-old woman, who had been in psychiatric hospital since the age of 17. Her diagnosis was of schizoaffective disorder. She had a long history of physical assault by her mother and stepfather and had a child at 16, whom she had given up for adoption. This had led to depression and serious self-harm, including swallowing razors and batteries.

She had spent the majority of her life in non-secure psychiatric settings but at age 37, as she faced the harsh fact of not having a baby whom she would be allowed to keep, she had taken another woman's baby, in the village where the hospital was located. She took the baby to a local park and sat with her by the swings, singing lullabies. The mother had been talking to a friend, a few feet from the pram but when she turned around her baby had vanished.

After a few hours Lily had returned to the hospital, with the baby girl still in its pram, by which time a major police operation was in place. Distressed and confused, as she had wanted only to spend a few hours pretending she had her own baby, to 'find out what it felt like', she felt terrified by the possibility of being sent away from this open ward, and, in her anxious state, set fire to her room. Her self-harm subsequently escalated and her mood deteriorated. She became violent to others and on one occasion attacked a nurse who had tried to encourage her into a bath, screaming 'leave the little girl alone', before biting and hitting her.[1]

Unfortunately this type of assault, combined with the fears about her potential to take a baby again, and her escalating self-harm, meant that she was detained in hospital for a further 13 years. Although she had spent the majority of her adult life in psychiatric hospital, she had always been allowed freedom and leave. After this incident she was charged with abduction and admitted to a medium secure psychiatric unit.

The last three years of her admission to medium security were spent in a women-only ward, until she was finally released into a mixed-sex secure environment, when I began to work with her, for a further two years. When I met her she looked like a rag-doll, with a defeated, distant air and a distracted manner. She was rarely violent, but when she was, it was directed towards her own body by cutting and burning her skin.

---

1   I later understood this as a regression to her abuse in childhood, which she associated with times of vulnerability and ostensible acts of care such as being bathed. It was at those times that her mother would become fraught and enraged, impatient with her slowness or shyness, and the beatings would be worst. Lily's assault on this nurse showed that at significant times where she felt vulnerable and child-like she reverted to a primitive defence of dissociation and a violent attempt to get rid of intrusion.

She had requested this move to a mixed environment, which had shocked the professionals who worked with her. The assumption had long been that she needed protection from men, as she was well known for exchanging sexual favours for cigarettes, and had become pregnant twice during her admission to the adult psychiatric ward. She had these pregnancies terminated, leaving her deeply unsettled and unhappy, with guilt feelings that persecuted her for a long time after.

Lily engaged in psychotherapy with me for a two-year period on the mixed low secure ward but initially the sessions were filled with silences, as she struggled to put her feelings into words. We explored her dreams, and the recurrent dream images she brought were of being a fish on a hook, caught in waves in the ocean, swept along until she was found strangled in a fishing net, with men and women on the shore, oblivious to her and dancing. This recurrent image of the fish had many variations: sometimes there was a swimming pool and men fishing on the side, in a pond; at other times there were rivers, streams and brambles; more often she dreamt of wild and crashing waves as she, the fish, was almost buried in the sand and detritus.

Lily told me about her childhood, in memory fragments, half-remembered images, and through dreams and her associations to them. It emerged that she was the eldest child and only daughter of a woman who had herself been abandoned into a care home at age three. Her mother had been 16 when she was born and, Lily felt, hated her, though she was far kinder to her other children; two boys born when she was three and five years old. These boys were treated with a degree of concern and affection, while she was more often left to fend for herself, or asked to tend to them for her mother.

Her mother would lash out at her frequently, saying she was a 'devil child'. Lily, a scared and unhappy child, wet the bed frequently, and this was often the catalyst for a beating; in turn she became more anxious and angry, and even more likely to wet the bed. This was a powerful symbol of her lack of containment. Occasionally her mother was kind and attentive to her, particularly after a violent assault, when she seemed to feel guilty, but Lily became more and more withdrawn, and trusted only her younger brothers and father, who seemed an increasingly distant presence. She didn't talk to him about the physical assaults at home that were now more frequent and severe. She lost her capacity to speak altogether for a short time in secondary school, where, unsurprisingly, her neglected appearance and nervous manner led to bullying.

As the only girl in the family, Lily had been expected to help her mother with her brothers and would often miss school to attend to them while her mother 'rested'. Her father was a heavy drinker but kind to her and sometimes, on a weekend, would take all three of the children fishing with him. Lily remembered that she would sit by him and feel safe. She thought he knew about her mother's brutality and would give her extra affection, calling her his 'special little girl', and seeming to worry most about her, but she was not sure he knew, and did not feel she could tell him. Sadly he left the family when she was eight, after discovering Lily's mother was having an affair, and she only saw him a few times a year, suffering instead from physical abuse at the hands of her mother's new boyfriend as well as her mother.

Lily could not stand the neglect and cruelty to which she had been subjected and sought solace in sexual encounters with men from an early age, but her attempt to become the mother she longed for was not successful. Her sense of emptiness and need stayed with her as she grew up and she longed for a baby who could help her to feel full and whole, and who would love her. As for so many other women the wish for a baby was a hope to have a loving creature inside of her, a source of affection and an affirmation of self-worth. Dinora Pines (1993) vividly describes the many unconscious fantasies of pregnancy that are discordant with the actual reality of childbirth, where a mother is not the recipient of love and care but must instead tend to the needs of a vulnerable, helpless and demanding infant.

Lily admitted that her early days with her baby girl, before she was taken into care, had been frightening, and she had found the baby's crying intolerable. She had wanted to hurt her, and this too had been terrifying, making her think that she would actually become her own brutal mother. Losing her baby into care, while something of a relief, was also a huge blow, leaving her feeling bereft and guilty.

She had taken the baby girl after rehearsing this scenario in fantasy for some weeks, following a distressing time in hospital when a trusted staff nurse had left the unit to have her own baby. Lily told me that she had wanted to 'share' the pregnancy with this nurse, and had hoped to be allowed to baby-sit. In her mind they had become like sisters. Her conscious fantasy was that she would learn to look after a baby and then make contact with this nurse, proving to her that she could be trusted. Unconsciously the aggression and envy she felt towards the nurse who had left her to have her own baby was enacted in relation to the mother of the baby she stole. She found this almost impossible to articulate but admitted too that she had, in a sense, enjoyed the fuss that her calm few hours with the baby had created. It seemed that she had little sense of this baby, or indeed any infant, as a subjective and individual being, with a bond with her mother that separation could damage. In the light of her own early experiences, her difficulty in imagining a baby's state of mind and empathising with its distress is not surprising (Newman and Sevenson 2005).

She had little sense of her own mind, and her own separate identity outside of being the unwanted girl who had tended to her mother's needs and demands, and who would suddenly, unpredictably, be beaten and hurt. Although she didn't actually harm the infant she had taken, it was difficult to know what would have happened if she had not been discovered, or if the baby had become inconsolable and shattered her fragile defences through crying. It is likely that Lily would then have felt persecuted by these cries, and could have become violent, either in desperation or retaliation (de Zulueta 1991).

THERAPEUTIC ENGAGEMENT

I felt that therapy with her was like working with a wounded animal that could be coaxed into the safety of a therapeutic home only gradually. She could barely sustain eye contact for more than a few seconds and her eyes followed my hands. She stammered and stared downward, seemed to lose focus altogether and related memories and thoughts as if still dreaming. In time she became able to talk about her index offence, but only at one remove as if someone else had taken the baby and she had been an observer.

I came to understand the recurrent images of fishing, and its significance for her, to symbolise the presence of a warm and loving person, her father, but also her own identification with something that was confusing and unpredictable, his failure to be protective and reliable. This was expressed in her feeling that she was like the fish who was hooked and left, flailing and flopping in the bracken. She would then be deserted and forgotten in some of the dreams, or half dead, watching from a distance as men and women danced together. The peaceful quality of her time with her father and brothers, and the terror of leaving this calm activity to return home, where her mother, often drunk, would be volatile and frightening, was embodied in the fish, whose abrupt removal from the water would mean its death.

In her need to preserve her father as a safe object, Lily had to 'forget' about his capacity to do harm towards his wife, her mother, of which she had been half aware. In later years her mother, who had by this time left Lily's stepfather, confided in her that she knew what she had done to her was wrong, and she had taken out her anger on her, but that Lily's father, the loving man so gentle to Lily, had often been cruel to her. Her mother explained she felt it was intolerable and that she had to get rid of that feeling. She did not explain why she continued to be violent to Lily when she had a new partner, who joined her in the assaults. She had used Lily as her poison container (de Mause 1990), the receptacle into which she could pour her own unbearable feelings and temporarily feel freed from them.

Lily described her sense of fear on the women's unit, feeling she was being punished for a sexual crime, connected with her terminations of pregnancy. She believed she was kept away from men because of what she might do to them, not because they might harm her.

The sense of danger that she carried inside her was heightened in the presence of so many women and she felt that she would drown in this sea. In contrast her father had allowed her to sit with him, on the banks, on solid ground.

Significantly, while she was able to tolerate visits from her mother, and to begin to understand her mother's perspective on why she had maltreated her, she also began regular, more frequent visits to her father, who though elderly and in poor health remained a supportive and kind figure. For many years after her mother's disclosures of his violence, and his withdrawal from the family, Lily had sealed herself off from contact with him and in her early 30s had begun to see him only a few times a year. By the end of therapy she was visiting him twice a month, and found this time precious.

Her brothers were loyal to her, inviting her to their houses on special occasions, but busy with their own wives and children, so this offered her a bittersweet experience, of being offered glimpses of home and family, and made welcome, but knowing that she herself would not be able to achieve this kind of stability. The dream images of the beautiful couples dancing while she watched, not human, not able to engage in reproductive intercourse, were often in my mind when I met with Lily. One of the central tasks for her, it seemed to me, was to be able to re-engage with her sexual self, and develop loving intimate relationships where she felt safe.

TRANSFER FROM MIXED-SEX TO WOMEN'S UNIT

With Lily's background in mind, would a women-only unit necessarily be the best place for her? And if so, what were the dangers of such a pattern being replicated? Lily experienced the women's unit as a frightening and claustrophobic environment and tended to avoid all the other patients, but trusted a few of the staff members, particularly those least likely to intrude or make demands.

On the women's unit she avoided other females, and formed a particularly strong bond with an older male charge nurse, with whom she could be seen sitting, infrequently saying anything. She would be found in a corner of a room, next to him, with her arms folded, looking into the distance, or engrossed in one of the many Sudoku puzzles that seemed to both distract her and protect her from engagement with others. It seemed to me that this was akin to her fishing outings with her father, where she could sit by him, but without too much intimate contact, engaged in activity and looking onto the river.

Lily considered the attempt to protect her, to place her within a female world, to be a form of punishment. It is possible that at unconscious level, in contrast to the conscious aim of protection, the decision was one designed to keep Lily's sexuality at bay, unable either to be used by others or revealed as a force in its own right, with procreative capacities.

It is this aspect of single-sex segregation that is difficult to explore in a climate that considers the notion of mixed-sex treatment inevitably to be dangerous and irresponsible. In one way the establishment of women-only units can be seen as a paternalistic and defensive response to the perceived problem of sexuality amongst psychiatric patients.

It also conceptualises women in intimate proximity to one another, as located in a necessarily healthier, safer, and more empowering place than a mixed-sex setting, which seems to ignore the impact of destructive dynamics that can take hold within such systems.

When considering Lily's index offence, and the concern it generated in terms of future risk to the community, her punishment/treatment of being moved to an all-female unit assumes many symbolic functions. It demonstrates the sense in which she was seen as the equivalent of the crone, or wicked witch in a fairy tale, drawn to steal and ultimately destroy the innocent offspring of good people. This danger must be confined to a safe and far-away land. She was therefore exiled from the land of ordinary families altogether and sent to a locked place where there was no possibility of reproductive sexuality.

Was she being sentenced to life in a sexless haven, a nunnery, or a women's prison, like a kind of witch's coven? The conflicting motivations in her crime, at once both ordinary and desperate, at the same time frightening and malicious, were mirrored in the confusion about how and where she should best be treated.

Her eventual treatment within a women-only medium secure unit also put me in mind of Hamlet's entreaty to Ophelia, after she confesses her love for him – she must be banished altogether and prevented from procreating, as to do so would be to reproduce more sinners, implying that she has a sexual voracity that can't be tamed:

Get thee to a nunnery! Why wouldst thou be a
breeder of sinners?… Go thy ways to a nunnery.

Hamlet, Act 3, Scene 1, 114–121

Hamlet's speech here has been variously interpreted, both as a plea to Ophelia to take herself and her errant sexuality away to a convent and as an insulting command to go to a brothel where she can cavort with other prostitutes. The irony of this pun on nunnery is that the ostensible haven for celibate women is in fact a place of prostitution, of sexuality used coldly for profit and the satisfaction of lust.

Lily's recurrent image of being caught and left, like the helpless, trapped fish, floundering in an entangled net, encapsulated her experience of being in the single-sex unit, where she felt she would linger and die. She longed for contact with the one secure adult in her life, her father, or another man who could replace him. This was impossible here and so she was left to pine, and watch others together, the heterosexual couples she saw in her dreams on beaches, and the nursing staff she would see laughing and joking with one another.

As Aiyegbusi (2004) powerfully argues, there is great potential for women-only units to offer reparative attachment experiences, provided that staff can tolerate and make sense of the repeated attacks and other communications they receive. In order to achieve this, staff of all disciplines and grades are expected to engage in regular training, supervision and reflective practice (staff support) where attachment principles are explained and difficult countertransference experiences can be processed, rather than being enacted:

Patients are trying to live with overwhelming emotional pain and project this into staff through various communications such as self injury, very direct sexualized communications, physical assaults and vicious personalized attacks…the unconscious hope is that the nursing staff can do something positive with the communication. (Aiyegbusi 2004)

However, for some women, whose early experiences of maternal abuse and neglect have been very severe, it is possible that this environment will be experienced as cruel, tantalising, and ultimately unmanageable, even where the staff have been highly trained and are sensitive to these difficulties. The need to have maternal care, apparently on offer, and the pain of its deprivation is so intense that the women feel compelled to pervert and destroy the care that is offered. They can find the situation of competing with other women for care and attention unbearable and rates of self-harm may escalate, as this becomes a currency of communication. In turn, managing high rates of self-harm places tremendous emotional strain on those staff members who are there to prevent, treat and understand it (Motz 2009).

Other female patients shy away from maternal care and its intensity, seeking a less demanding emotional engagement in wards that also house men. Some may even feel more sexually threatened by close proximity to female patients, particularly those who have abused children sexually. One woman who had been sexually abused by her own mother, and her aunt, found that sleeping next door to a female sex offender was terrifying, and she ran away from the ward at the first opportunity, eventually being found under a railway bridge, in a dishevelled state. Her levels of self-harm escalated seriously when she was returned to the ward. These attacks on her body were symbolically assaults on others, and a concrete reproach to those tasked with caring for her. It revealed the extent of her fear, anger and wish to be removed from this ward and taken to a place where she felt safe.

An unconscious wish in the establishment of women-only units is that sexual perversion and violence will safely be located outside the ward, in the male patients. This was not the felt experience of this woman, or of several others with her history. The woman who had abused children entrusted to her care was seen as far worse than paedophilic men, and being locked up with her day and night was a terrifying reminder of inescapable maternal abuse, although staff reassured the other women that they were vigilant and would protect them. While these reassurances addressed their conscious fears to a limited extent, the unconscious fantasies of being invaded and hurt by this predatory woman remained.

I MADE YOU TO FIND ME

To examine how toxic, destructive relationships can develop within women-only units, despite the best intentions of those who design and work in them, it is essential to consider the dynamics of maternal deprivation and abuse and the trajectories these create. Women in secure care predominantly have histories of abuse, neglect, time in local authority care and attempts in adolescence to blank out the pain through drug and alcohol use. Their early lives are often characterised by maternal abuse and neglect and a cycle of re-victimisation with partners, as well as frantic attempts to become pregnant themselves (see also Chapter 1).

The hope of women-only units is that through 'relational security' dangerous behaviour will be reduced. Furthermore, through secure attachments between care staff and the patients, and between the patients themselves, the capacity to form healthy relationships will develop. The model of care within the women-only units is based on attachment research and attempts to take account of the deeply disturbed early experiences of many of the women, whose impact has been felt throughout their lives. This hope can itself reflect some denial of the damage that women can do to their own offspring, and to one another, indeed a denial of female violence.

The idealisation of motherhood is a powerful blinding force that can make the notion of a single-sex refuge appear benign and welcome, when, in fact, it may have powerful associations for these women of captivity and maternal abuse (see also Chapter 10). 'Mothering, whether in the home, or on the hospital floor, is a much more common route to power for psychopathic women than is commerce or sex' (Pearson 1998).

In her poem 'The Double Image', Anne Sexton (1928–1974), who suffered from serious depression and eventually committed suicide, describes her own early years with her daughter Joyce, alongside the difficult relationship with her own mother, who never forgives her for her attempted suicide, and is herself ill with cancer. The poem is written to Joyce and is in her first collection of poems, *To Bedlam and Part Way Back*, from 1960 (Sexton 1999; emphasis added):

> …I remember we named you Joyce
> so we could call you Joy.
> You came like an awkward guest
> that first time, all wrapped and moist
> and strange at my heavy breast.

I needed you. I didn't want a boy,
only a girl, a small milky mouse
of a girl, already loved, already loud in the house
of herself. We named you Joy.
I, who was never quite sure
about being a girl, needed another
life, another image to remind me.
And this was my worst guilt; you could not cure
or soothe it. I made you to find me.

In this beautiful but chilling description of maternal narcissism (and depression) Sexton reveals her true wish in having her daughter, and its futility, foreshadowing the eventual outcome. She remains uncured. In fact, she finally left both her daughters through her suicide at age 46, and before that she frequently had to leave them to be admitted to hospital for treatment of her depression. She describes her guilt in her poetry, having taken up writing as part of her therapy. Her daughter Lynda later wrote in her autobiography that Sexton had sexually assaulted her in her childhood, as well as physically abusing both her and her sister.

As Welldon (1988) has shown, the forum of mothering is a means by which a disturbed and maltreated mother can (unconsciously) wreak revenge on her own children, and repeat the destructive patterns of her past. The intergenerational transmission of abuse and neglect is striking; resounding through her treatment of her children are echoes of the mother's own childhood.

BEREFT MEN AND WOMEN

One of the consequences of single-sex wards in forensic mental health settings is that social contact between men and women is greatly reduced and that even where therapeutic meetings were anticipated the reality is often that virtual ghettos are formed. The single-sex units serve as traditional custodial environments in which the unacceptable elements of society are housed, and, most importantly the anxiety about their potential reproduction is reduced. Like the psychiatric hospitals of old, men and women are kept apart, and their meetings, if they happen at all, are strictly monitored, reminiscent of the traditional dances in high secure hospital where male and female patients mixed for a short, controlled period of time.

In the new single-sex environments even the dances are gone, and yet, once there is a 'step down' to lower security, the women can once again live with male patients, and now the potential exists again to form the very relationships that the women-only units were designed to exterminate. The logic of this is fuzzy, but it seems there is an unconscious equation with dangerousness and sexuality such that patients in high and medium secure settings are unsafe to live together, even in separated bays, but the closer they come to the community, to, as it were, regaining human status, the safer they are to be together. This leads to confusing inconsistencies whereby people discharged from high secure settings are seen as magically transformed, and can establish relationships with one another that are condoned. It is as if their vulnerability and capacity to damage one another has been forgotten.

I have worked closely with the men on wards where the women had left and been witness to the mourning they experienced, not for sexual partners, but for the people who had imparted some sense of liveliness and emotionality into the ward, serving as mother figures as well as friends. One man said 'the whole place now felt dead', that the women were 'the life and soul of the place'. Others described their real fear of being left only with men, and a sense that the presence of the women had prevented violence, reminding the men to take care of others and manage their own impulses. Their presence was felt to be protective, and to reduce the risk of violence. The affectionate relationships that had existed sometimes included physical touching and 'cuddling' but both the men who were left and the women who had moved insisted this had been consensual. The taboo of sexuality in psychiatric patients was not eradicated as homosexual abuse and coercion continued to exist, but perhaps this was even more difficult to face and manage, so had to go underground. Several men expressed the fear that they would turn increasingly to female staff to meet all their needs for social and emotional, or even sexual, contact with women. There was an overwhelming sense of loss.

In their study of women in single-sex secure accommodation, Mezey, Hassell and Bartlett (2005) found only partial support for the assumption that women patients in secure psychiatric settings will feel safer if they are segregated from the male patients. They concluded that:

> Although most women patients in the segregated units felt safe, many of them nevertheless stated that they would prefer to be in a mixed-

sex ward. Gender segregation was associated in many women's minds with prison and was regarded as 'abnormal'. Any increased protection that such settings might afford was outweighed by the reputation of women-only units as punitive and stigmatising. Moreover, some women patients said that their sense of safety would be increased if there were more male patients and staff on the ward. Women are detained in secure psychiatric settings because of their risk of violence and aggression. It should therefore not be surprising if, even when these women are segregated from the men, the ward environment may remain disturbed and at times dangerous. (2005, p.582)

My own discussions with women who had left the mixed-sex unit revealed similar themes of loss and bereavement, as well as fear about proximity to the other women, and the potential for bullying and intimidation within the ward. Several reported feeling imprisoned and held captive, while others felt as invisible and helpless in this new surrounding as they had on the male ward. They welcomed improved access to therapies, but the difficulty of facing so many women, and living in such an emotionally intense environment, was a repeated theme. One woman said it felt like she was in 'a hall of mirrors' and was constantly confronted with distorted reflections of herself and her own mother.

For some women the single-sex unit was the safe haven they desperately needed. Women who had been sexually abused by men within their family particularly valued freedom from encounters with male patients.

CONCLUSION: RELATIONAL SECURITY FOR ALL

The provision of therapeutic wards where privacy is valued, protection offered, but total segregation is not the norm would offer both men and women safety, security and psychological care rather than simply containment: this may be the compromise that is required. While segregating men and women at the highest level of security may still be necessary, at all lower stages a mixed therapeutic environment, with separate and protected bedrooms for each gender, may in fact prove to be more helpful and less toxic than single-sex treatments.

Single-sex units can have great value but can also be seen as a defence against anxiety. This is anxiety related to the sexuality and potential procreativity of forensic patients, and a denial of the violence, aggression and perversion of which women as well as men are capable.

The central question is whether it is possible to combine separate sleeping spaces for men and women, where privacy and dignity are maintained, while still providing a therapeutic milieu in which the psychological needs of vulnerable and dangerous men and women will be met. The physical separation of men and women, while sometimes desirable, is not a universal solution for all; it is not always in the patients' best interests and if prescribed without careful consideration could simply reflect the primitive psychic defence of splitting, offering a concrete solution to the complex problem of how to house dangerous states of mind (Scanlon and Adlam 2006).[2]

---

2   One NHS trust in Whittington expresses the following in relation to general hospital wards, but it would be possible to extend the principles to mental health units too:

Same Sex Accommodation – Safeguarding your privacy and dignity
Maintaining privacy and dignity for our patients is a key priority and over the past year we have invested over £1.2 million to improve the 'patient experience' on our wards.

      One of our most important actions has been to ensure that men and women staying in our hospital do not have to share their accommodation with patients of the opposite sex. Being comfortable in your surroundings is a key part of maintaining dignity and our Trust Board is fully committed to eradicating mixed sex accommodation.

      In January 2009, the Secretary of State for Health announced an intensive drive to all but eliminate mixed sex accommodation. Hospital Trusts are now required to publish a 'declaration of compliance' stating whether or not they are able to declare the virtual elimination of mixed sex accommodation and its continued delivery. We have carried out a ward improvement programme to help address this. To date we have refurbished six wards across the Trust to ensure they comply with the single sex standard.

      The work we have undertaken means that our patients on mixed sex wards can now be accommodated in single sex bays, with dedicated bathroom and toilet facilities. Arranging patients' accommodation in this way (using single sex bays rather than single sex wards) means we can still provide the specialist clinical care patients need.

REFERENCES

Aiyegbusi, A. (2004) 'Thinking under Fire.' In N. Jeffcote and T. Watson (eds) *Working Therapeutically with Women in Secure Mental Health*. London: Jessica Kingsley Publishers.

Bland, J., Mezey, G. and Dolan, B. (1999) 'Special women, special needs: a descriptive study of female special hospital patients.' *Journal of Forensic Psychiatry 10*, 1, 34–45.

Coid, J. *et al.* (2003) (unpublished) *A Study of Gender Differences in a Household Population Sample.*

de Mause, L. (1990) 'The history of child assault.' *Journal of Psychohistory 18*, 1, 1–29.

Department of Health (2002) *Women's Mental Health: Into the Mainstream. Strategic Development of Mental Health Care for Women*. London: Department of Health.

de Zulueta, F. (1991) *From Pain to Violence: The Traumatic Roots of Destructiveness*. Chichester: John Wiley.

Mezey, G., Hassell, Y. and Bartlett, A. (2005) 'Safety of women in mixed-sex and single-sex medium secure units: staff and patient perceptions.' *British Journal of Psychiatry 187*, 579–582.

Motz, A. (ed.) (2009) *Managing Self Harm: Psychological Perspectives*. Hove: Brunner-Routledge.

Newman, L. and Sevenson, C. (2005) 'Ghosts in the nursery: parenting and borderline personality disorder.' *Clinical Child Psychology and Psychiatry 10*, 3, 385–394.

Pearson, P. (1998) *When She Was Bad*. London: Virago.

Pines, D. (1993) *A Woman's Unconscious Use of Her Body*. London: Virago.

Scanlon, C. and Adlam, J. (2006) 'Housing "unhoused minds" – inter-personality disorder in the organisation?' *Journal of Housing, Care and Support 9*, 3, 9–14.

Sexton, A. (1999) *Anne Sexton: The Complete Poems*. London: Houghton Mifflin.

Welldon, E. (1988) *Mother, Madonna, Whore: The Idealisation and Denigration of Motherhood*. New York: Guilford Press.

Chapter 8

ANNIHILATING THE OTHER
Forensic Aspects of Organisational Change

Martin Wrench

In this chapter Martin Wrench describes how the particular milieu of the Henderson Hospital was 'shot by both sides', succumbing to both 'friendly' as well as more obviously hostile fire. In contrast to Neeld and Clarke, whose chapter described the work of a unit now closed, to Motz, who looked at the reconfiguration of a whole sector, and to Taylor, whose context is the work of an adapted therapeutic community that is 'still standing' under fire, Wrench now takes us into the detail of the dénouement of a therapeutic community. He offers an analysis of its closure, looking not just at assaults upon it from outside, but also from within, and he uses sociological and systems-psychodynamic models of understanding to capture the complex processes involved.

INTRODUCTION

When I first presented the paper on which this chapter is based in December 2007, I was writing in the context of the pending closure of the Henderson Hospital, a residential therapeutic community for people with personality disorder that had been open for sixty years and had established an international reputation almost from the time it opened to the point at which commissioning changes in the NHS and wider societal changes threatened its existence. As someone who had worked in forensic services and had consulted to teams and organisations for many years, and as a staff member passionately committed to the Therapeutic Community model of treatment, I wanted to gain an understanding of why it and other residential therapeutic communities were under threat.

The opportunity to write this paper gave me the impetus to gain a clearer understanding of why the service was threatened and what confluence of societal and human impulses was contributing to its probable closure. Of course, in the natural order of things, institutions close and humans die. In the latter case, except in times of war, rarely at the hands of another and in the case of institutions it is true that they can often outgrow their usefulness and become redundant. The Henderson was not seemingly an institution that had outlived its usefulness since patients, or residents, as they were known, continued to benefit and a year before its eventual closure there was a waiting list for admission, and a set of positive independent research evaluations were about to be published. Clearly, clinicians and service users still valued the treatment. However, we were also aware that changes were necessary if it was to survive in the NHS marketplace and there were working groups in the organisation exploring ways to change or adapt in relation to emergent tension between the needs of the residents and the demands of commissioners. Ultimately, though, my sense was that, whatever efforts we made to adapt to prevailing conditions and demands, the Henderson was to be killed off, indeed murdered, for being out of step with the modernising and homogenising culture of the NHS to which it represented something inimical. So in the manner of anyone who feels threatened, in danger of serious harm or, as in this case, who wants to protect an organisation, I went in search of the source of the violence and for a perpetrator or perpetrators who could be held to account for this prospective crime; a perpetrator whose motivation could be understood, even if this understanding could not prevent the crime.

When I joined in 1999, the Henderson with Department of Health funding was in the process of supporting the development of two new services that were set up to replicate the Henderson model of treatment: Main House in Birmingham and Webb House in Crewe (Norton 2006). How was it that the residential therapeutic community was going from boom to bust in such a short space of time? (Webb House closed in 2006, the Henderson in 2008 and Main House in 2010.) What changes were occurring in society that might explain this and was there a relationship between the nature of the work, treating severe personality disorder, and the demise of the organisations treating them? At the time of the presentation I identified three 'perpetrators' that were threatening the Henderson's existence. These were, first of all, what Zygmunt Bauman (2000) has described as 'liquid modernity'; second, the denial and fear of feeling in modern welfare and healthcare brilliantly defined and explored in Cooper and Lousada's (2005) *Borderline Welfare: Feeling and Fear of Feeling in Modern Welfare*; and lastly the increasing ascendency of the internal market in the NHS, as represented through commissioning bodies or individual commissioners, which can be understood to have its roots in liquid modernity and borderline welfare.

My view at the time of the presentation in December 2007 was that the perpetrators of this offence were personified and embodied by the market-driven, liquidly modern exponents of borderline welfare who may have had little or no understanding of what determined their actions. However, a question that I did not consider until a few months after the closure was to ask what the Henderson as an organisation might have contributed to its own demise. Now more than three years after the closure it is possible to reflect with more objectivity on the possibility, indeed the likelihood, that the borderline, antisocial and narcissistic difficulties that these services were designed to treat also affected the organisation's capacity to respond effectively to the forces arraigned against it: that there may have been some propensity for self-harm in an organisation that could not protect itself or mobilise sufficiently to adjust to new and challenging circumstances. I shall explore further the extent to which the victim may have failed to protect itself, or invited attack, after discussion of what I see to be the attackers' characteristics and 'motivation'.

LIQUID MODERNITY AND THE END OF 'THE COMMUNITY'

In *Liquid Modernity* Bauman (2000) discusses Marx' and Engels' reference to 'melting the solids', those entrenched impediments to progress that had become stagnant or ossified. Bauman states that Marx and Engels were intent on replacing the older 'solid order' with new and improved solidarity; replacing the old class structures and caste loyalties with what Weber termed an 'instrumental rationality' presided over by economic and historical determinism. If history did not work out quite as Marx or Engels envisaged it, economics, as a result of what we might call an 'instrumental irrationality' in the form of liquid capitalism and its technological innovations, has indeed determined the main narrative of post-modernity where the ever-increasing speed of adaptation and communication has 'melted the solids' to the point where we inhabit 'liquid life'. Liquid life is a fundamentally insecure condition where individuals have to endlessly adapt to new challenges and cannot depend on experience or knowledge acquired over time because what we know now rapidly becomes obsolete. One of the key elements of liquid modernity is the presence of 'zombie' categories or institutions – for example the family, class and neighbourhood – all of which are stripped of life and meaning but continue in zombie forms that bear little relation to how they were understood by past generations.

The same can be said of our understanding of 'community', which in Bauman's view has become a zombie category. Bauman dedicates a chapter to Community in *Liquid Modernity* and states that the word has been used more indiscriminately and emptily as it has become harder to find what sociologically might be considered a community in real life. This has been demonstrably the case with regard to so-called 'Care in the Community' where the solid institution of the mental hospital, with all its faults and failings, has been largely replaced by something far less solid and containing for those in need of help. One consequence is that patients can now be treated using Community Treatment Orders (CTOs), three words that in combination seem to my mind to destabilise each other. One is left wondering how we can understand community in this context or on whose behalf and in whose community is treatment being ordered or provided.

In a similar way, at the time of writing, the UK government's attempt to build the Big Society does indeed seem a hollow, empty attempt to recreate a sense of community in a society where for the past 30 years or more we have been encouraged to believe that the individual is paramount. The notion that 'we are all in it together and we will mend our broken society – together' (www.conservatives.com) as David Cameron stated in response to the so-called shopping riots of 2011 is, regrettably, just that – a notion – and one that falsifies differences in class, mobility, power and economic status.

Although only available to residents for a year, the Henderson was a community where staff and residents were engaged in a joint enterprise of peer learning where disturbances in 'groupishness', to use Bion's (1961) rather inelegant term, were explored and to varying degrees addressed by focusing on the daily running of the community as a 'living/learning experience'. It could be characterised as a place where people profoundly lacking in solidity, a sense of a coherent, agentive self, could develop, through being with and working alongside others, a more coherent sense of themselves: a container where residents (and staff) could attain some solidity and substance in a society where everything was becoming more liquid (Adlam and Scanlon 2009). Research conducted at Henderson Hospital indicated the benefit of this treatment in terms both of symptom reduction post-treatment (Dolan *et al.* 1997) and a substantial cost-offset in relation to the reduction in health, social care and criminal justice involvement in the year following treatment (Dolan *et al.* 1996) – results that continued to be evidenced even up to its last days (Norton 2009). Such evidence, while allowing initially for the development of two more therapeutic communities, did not count for much when the combined forces of liquid modernity, the internal market in healthcare and borderline welfare resulted in an irresistible flood of target-driven modernisation and homogenisation.

LIQUID LIFE MEETS BORDERLINE WELFARE

To the list of zombie categories can be added many of our social institutions including the welfare state itself (Cooper and Lousada 2005; see also Chapter 9). These are for the most part no longer solid entities or concepts. NHS Trusts are just one example of how post-modern organisations adapt, change and swallow each other up with remarkable ease and rapidity and with little apparent regard to the effect this has on the welfare or well-being of staff or patients. The term 'Foundation Hospital' or 'Trust' may create the impression of something solidly built, but such entities may prove to be as ephemeral as the 'Mental Health Trusts' that preceded them. Furthermore, as Abadi (2003) and other authors have made clear, we now live in a networked world where interdependency and community, for example the online community or the worldwide web, have a fluidity and decentred quality that, for better and for worse, bears little relation to the solidity and enduring nature of how previous generations experienced either communities or organisations.

Similarly, Cooper and Dartington (2004) argue that there was a post-war national consensus underpinning the setting up of the welfare state that was securely housed within a single ministry; over time, however, this focus has been lost and the presence of different ministries with often conflicting agendas and priorities has resulted in the absence of a coherent narrative with regard to the underlying principles of welfare provision. Faced with these conditions, Cooper and Lousada (2005) ask, 'Must we embrace instability of mind to be capable of working with such conditions of life? Or can "containment" assume some new meaning and psychic location?' Their diagnosis of what has gone wrong largely bears on the breakdown of trust between those in government and those delivering and receiving welfare and health provision; a consequence of what they refer to as 'anxious regulation'. In this 'borderline' world providers are not to be trusted and must be regulated and overseen, with the result they become anxious and propitiatory, more intent on avoiding criticism than uncovering truth. A further consequence is that the 'other', whether those setting the targets and regulatory framework, or the provider or receiver of services, is perceived as a threat rather than as participant in an enterprise of mutual benefit, as part of the social contract (Rustin 2004).

At this point the social contract itself is now a zombie category hastened in its undead existence by the Friedmanite and Thatcherite espousal and implementation of market capitalism: the privatising of what was previously the public sphere. This privatising process is one that successive governments have adhered to with little apparent consideration of the impact on those it affects. One consequence of privatisation and the predominance of market forces is that an illusion has to be sustained, in the publicity that supports it, that there is only 'good news' (Cooper and Lousada 2005). In this world of 'Goodthink' (Orwell 1948), any bad news or failure, if such thoughts can be entertained even fleetingly, has to be the fault of the 'other' who is deemed insufficiently engaged or in line with regulatory principles and the dominant narrative of positive results. So despite service closures and staff losses, everything is going well, 'service improvement' targets are being met, patients are 'recovering' (Scanlon and Adlam 2010) and everyone is entitled to be a member of the 'Foundation Trust' even though such membership offers only the vaguest of benefits, little if any influence and a spurious sense of belonging. As a consequence, complexity and what are described as 'ambivalent structures of feeling' (Cooper and Lousada 2005) are simplified in futile attempts to avoid anxiety and uncertainty.

The conditions under borderline welfare and liquid modernity with the limited opportunity they provide for depth of engagement and complexity or ambivalence of feeling were, to my mind, inimical to the therapeutic community that had developed at the Henderson and its 'offshoots' (Wrench and Menzies 2006) over 60 years. There 'bad news' was an integral part of the work as residents struggled to share the experience of the trauma, abuse, neglect and insecurity that had characterised their early years and given shape to the emotional, relational and behavioural problems that had brought them there. The Henderson provided a container where residents could experiment with new and less self-defeating ways of managing hurt and distress and develop a different experience of the 'other' who in the past may have been only a source of threat, harm or neglect (see Chapters 1, 4 and 12).

Cooper and Lousada (2005) describe how welfare provision is problematic and fraught with complex and ambivalent feelings in no small part because 'welfare exists to provide care and services to the stranger or "other" and the stranger is often as likely to provoke hostility as compassion.' In the Henderson, where the residents had the most votes in relation to who was invited to join the community, the issue of otherness had to be confronted, explored and addressed from the off. Was this person seeking admission potentially to harm one of us or might his or her 'otherness' pose a threat to the integrity of the community? Is this person able to use the treatment provided by the therapeutic community and can he or she tolerate us and can we live with him or her? Underneath, however, may lie the threat of annihilation posed by too much proximity. For the person seeking admission, the fear perhaps of being damaged or overwhelmed by the 'other' or 'others' and, for those assessing the applicant, similar fears of being engulfed or overwhelmed, may also have been elicited. This dread of too much proximity on the one hand or the danger of separation and abandonment on the other hand is elaborated in Glasser's (1979) description of the 'core complex' as a primitive level of functioning where the individual seeks merger with the 'other' in blissful or idealised union. The danger is that associated with the desired state is intense fear and anxiety about losing one's identity or sense of self, of being engulfed or annihilated by the 'other'. In order to resist being overwhelmed or threatened with annihilation the individual may act violently towards the 'other' to kill off the threat by killing off the initially desired or needed 'other'.

In the later stages of the Henderson's life the issue of commissioners as an embodiment of the 'other', who would either assist in continuing to bring life or were intent on closing it down and killing it off, was active in the minds of the staff. Commissioners were at times viewed as insatiable in their demands. The service had to be modified, treatment episodes shortened, residents should no longer select each other; in their view it was a commissioning, not a clinical or evidential, decision about who was treated and in what ways. The view seemed to be 'change or die' but the difficulty was posed in relation to a master-servant or indeed victim-perpetrator dynamic where the commissioners, with Trust managers, determined what was needed and what needed changing without appreciating the damage it would do to the treatment model or without taking into account the accumulated evidence that supported its efficacy and effectiveness.

Staff and residents *were* prepared to adapt or make changes but too much intrusion from those who had little understanding of personality disorder and the modus operandi of the Henderson was considered detrimental to effective treatment and was also feared and resented. Managers in the Trust showed little appetite for keeping the service open unless a partner organisation could share or own the financial risk. We were courted briefly by some other organisations but no marriage was proposed. It seemed from how these private and voluntary organisations engaged with us that any such marriage would result in the annihilation of the Henderson as anything other than a brand. Its core identity would have been compromised to an unacceptable degree. Their approach too, though initially welcome, seemed inimical to the highly developed collaborative ethos between staff and residents on which the entire work of the Henderson was premised.

These organisations seemed products of borderline welfare inherently unable to address the complex feelings engendered in relation to the 'other' and as an organisation the Henderson was threatened either by annihilation through engulfment or death. Unlike a patient operating at the level of the core complex the Henderson did not have the self-preservative option of killing off the 'other', although the wish to do so was active in both residents and staff and openly expressed in groups and in staff meetings. At a more mature level of functioning, staff and residents with support from ex-residents and other concerned clinicians joined together in campaigning for the Henderson's survival.

The relationship with managers in the Trust was complex: were they the 'enemy within', aligned with commissioners that by and large we felt did not understand or respect the work we were doing or the evidence base for it, or could they save the Henderson by gaining the support of the Trust Board in keeping the Henderson alive?

From my experience of the closure process and with the benefit of three years' subsequent reflection it is all too apparent to me that the management was unwilling to support the Henderson but the managers involved may have a very different perception of their role and intentions.

THE IMPACT OF TRAUMA AND THE NATURE OF THE WORK

It is important to bear in mind that the severity of the disorder that was being treated at the Henderson was also having an impact on the therapeutic community's relationship with itself and others. The Henderson during my time working there had been described as both the Trust's jewel in the crown and its white elephant: it was admired but also envied and resented, viewed as ahead of its time even after 60 years but also as outdated because of its age and working principles and practices.

Reflecting this there was perhaps a borderline disturbance operating in the organisation that made it difficult for the Henderson to be anything other than exceptional or worthless and impaired its capacity to find or maintain a balanced perspective. Antisocial and narcissistic features in the form of self-aggrandisement, self-harming and destructive behaviour were also a possible factor in the Henderson's management's failure to secure a future for the therapeutic community. As someone directly involved and aware of the attempts to secure a future, I feel confident in saying that the staff and the management team of which I was a member were not on an unconscious suicide mission to bring down the Henderson; nor so hostile to the Trust management or potential bids from other agencies as to reduce the possibility of survival through narcissistic arrogance. It is important to be alive, however, to the possibility that the Henderson was a disordered institution that related in a disordered way to the pressures it faced. Whatever the contribution of the staff, including myself, may have been to its closure, my view remains that the Henderson was closed, as much as for any other reason, because it had come to represent something threatening to the dissociative processes that sustain borderline welfare with its seeming denial of human distress and its reliance on Orwellian Goodthink. Everything currently in the NHS in relation to mental health seems to my mind to be to do with recovery and well-being, but trauma, hurt, violence and distress seem to have been deleted from the discourse relating to mental health (Scanlon and Adlam 2010). Is it any surprise if managers wedded to the discourse of recovery and cost-cutting would do little to enable the Henderson and its more complex and nuanced relation to distress and its causes (and to recovery) to survive?

In the *Guardian* obituary of the celebrated psychoanalyst Hanna Segal, she is quoted as follows in relation to global oppression: 'this expanding global empire, like all such things, has to be sustained through control of the media – and this is of necessity based on a series of lies. From the humane (and psychoanalytic) point of view we are led as citizens to struggle with the unending task of exposing lies for the preservation of sane humane values – this is our only hope' (*Guardian*

2011). My response to this quote, as it applies to mental health services, is that exposing half-truths rather than lies is the task. In some ways half-truths are more dangerous than outright mendacity. In more overt lying, at least the liar recognises what is being concealed and the threat posed by what needs to be hidden. Promoting a half-truth may be as much about an inability to recognise what is concealed as an attempt to hide something. The Henderson was able to contain and address the possibility of recovery but finding one's voice and a more secure sense of self required struggle and the possibility of pain, conflict and rejection as well as more positive thoughts, feelings and experiences and could not be achieved as an act of will or in response to societal prescriptions or injunctions. The fact had to be faced that not everyone gets better despite our best efforts, wishes or intentions. This possibility does not exist in a world of half-truths and it therefore becomes impossible to talk about or address failure. Killing off the institution that represents a more complex reality is a good price to pay for sustaining a collective and pain-free Panglossian fantasy that 'all is for the best in the best of all possible worlds' (Voltaire 1759).

A key word in the Segal quotation is *citizen*. Citizenship is a problematic concept and possibly also a zombie category. Borderline welfare as expressed by marketisation in the NHS denotes a breakdown in citizenship, as it places the market above the needs and wishes of the service user and the clinician – despite all the talk about such half truths as localism, the 'big society' and community values, and one's right to be a member of an NHS Trust. The reality or 'truth' seems to be that commissioners *do* determine what service users will receive, based upon economic analyses of incomplete NICE guidelines that limit or deny access to therapies for people with complex problems: often those that do not easily respond to cognitive behavioural therapy (CBT) or other brief interventions and so do not experience their access to psychological therapies as being improved (Scanlon and Adlam 2010). It is a feature of liquid modernity and borderline welfare that complexity and depth are replaced by surface and simplification. Baumann (2005) prefaces *Liquid Life* with a quote from Ralph Waldo Emerson: 'When skating over thin ice, our safety is in our speed.' Cooper and Dartington (2004) ask if, in the fluid world of 'negotiated interdependences', new possibilities for depth engagement may arise but they cannot conceive what in a fluid world might offer containment to sustain that level of engagement. At the time of writing the world economy is at risk of implosion because of the absence of containing structures. Money has gone virtual and has slipped the bounds of any container and as a result there is no rational economic instrumentality – just an ever-increasing number of phantom, zombie or junk instruments that can no longer perpetuate the illusion of endless growth and progress.

CHANGE OR DIE – FROM BOOM TO BUST

The Henderson and its offshoots (or grafts) were not allowed the chance to continue to adapt and change meaningfully because they were based on principles antithetical to the prevailing culture of quick and ready and painless solutions to all problems in the public and private sphere. In this climate change was never really an option because the changes that were requested kept changing with every new prospective partner or every new commissioning group or individual commissioner. It proved impossible to refine or re-define the therapeutic community at a time when the welfare state had acquired such borderline features, splitting off and denigrating the recipient of welfare and where the concept of community itself had become reduced to an empty slogan.

Bauman (2010) has stated that society can only be raised to the level of community if it protects all its members from the horror of exclusion, social redundancy and of being viewed as human waste. The Henderson was a community in no small part because it placed the value of the human above that of the market. It was a small organisation centred around changing peoples' lives and was and remains much loved by those whose lives were improved – it was also sometimes derided or hated by those it failed (and possibly also hated and derided by those who failed it?). The Henderson elicited passion, rarely indifference, and it allowed for the expression of painful and complex feelings by providing structure, containment and continuity over time. Containment, security and stability enable the individual to stand back and reflect on him or herself in relation to self and others. In a *Guardian* review of Cees Noteboom's collection of stories *The Foxes Come at Night*, Alberto Manguel comments on Noteboom forcing his readers to 'reflect on what is being said, and to take up their part in the work: for him literature is a collaborative effort.' Manguel contrasts the demands Noteboom places on the reader with his view that 'the stories we prefer must be told quickly, and allow for little pause and less reflection. Our preferred condition is foolishness.'

This foolishness, whether sought or imposed on us by liquid modernity and borderline welfare, has led to the simplification of the narrative relating to emotional and psychological distress and the seeming loss of the collaborative and communitarian ethos that informed the Henderson. Whether new sources of containment will arise that will allow for the re-emergence of nuanced, balanced and sophisticated forms of reflection, growth and change is hard to envisage but it is important that we continue to take up the challenge to engage with, reflect on and develop those elements in our culture that are at risk of annihilation because their otherness runs counter to the insidious notion that the difficulties, traumas and distress resulting from the human condition are ones that we can speedily recover from.

REFERENCES

Abadi, S. (2003) 'Between the frontier and the network: notes for a metapsychology of freedom.' *International Journal of Psychoanalysis 84*, 2, 221–234.

Adlam, J. and Scanlon, C. (2009) 'Disturbances of "groupishness"? Structural violence, refusal and the therapeutic community response to severe personality disorder.' *International Forum of Psychoanalysis 18*, 1, 23–29.

Bauman, Z. (2000) *Liquid Modernity.* Cambridge: Polity Press.

Bauman, Z. (2005) *Liquid Life.* Cambridge: Polity Press.

Bauman, Z. (2010) *Living on Borrowed Time: Conversations with Citlali Rovirosa-Madrazo.* Cambridge: Polity Press.

Bion, W.R. (1961) *Experiences in Groups.* London: Karnac.

Cooper, A. and Dartington, T. (2004) 'The vanishing organisation: organizational containment in a networked world.' In C. Huffington, D. Armstrong, W. Halton, L. Holye and J. Pooley (eds) *Working Below the Surface: the Emotional Life of Contemporary Organisations.* London: Karnac.

Cooper, A. and Lousada, J. (2005) *Borderline Welfare: Feeling and Fear of Feeling in Modern Welfare.* London: Karnac.

Dolan, B.M., Warren, F., Menzies, D. and Norton, K. (1996) 'Cost-offset following specialist treatment of severe personality disorders.' *The Psychiatrist 20*, 413–417.

Dolan, B. M., Warren, F. and Norton, K. (1997) 'Change in borderline symptoms one year after therapeutic community treatment for severe personality disorder.' *The British Journal of Psychiatry 171*, 249–279.

Glasser, M. (1979) 'Some Aspects of the Role of Aggression in the Perversions.' In I. Rosen (ed.) *Sexual Deviation.* Oxford: Oxford University Press.

Guardian (2008) 'Queen of Darkness.' 8 September 2008. Available at www.guardian.co.uk/science/2008/sep/08/psychology.healthandwellbeing, accessed on 2 February 2012.

Guardian (2011) 'Obituary: Hanna Segal.' 15 July 2011.

Norton, K. (2006) *Setting Up New Services in the NHS: 'Just Add Water!'* London: Jessica Kingsley Publishers.

Norton, K. (2009) 'Understanding failures of NHS policy implementation in relation to borderline personality disorder.' *Psychodynamic Practice 15*, 1, 25–40.

Orwell, G. (1948) *1984.* London: Secker and Warburg.

Rustin, M. (2004) 'Re-thinking audit and inspection.' *Soundings 64*, 86–107.

Scanlon, C. and Adlam, J. (2010) 'The *Recovery Model* or the modelling of a cover-up? On the creeping privatisation and individualisation of dis-ease and being-unwell-ness.' *Groupwork 20*, 3, 100–114 (Special Issue on Groupwork and Well-Being).

Voltaire (1759/1997) *Candide.* London: Penguin Books.

Wrench, M. and Menzies, D. (2006) 'Henderson Outreach Service Team: "Offshoot or graft?" *Mental Health Review 11*, 2, 174–185.

Chapter 9

HOW TO (ALMOST) MURDER A PROFESSION
The Unsolved Mystery of British Social Work

Andrew Cooper

In this chapter Andrew Cooper takes the case, not just of a singular milieu or sector caught in the crossfire, but of a whole profession under attack. He refers to processes of mourning as well as of murder. He vividly describes the persecution of the social workers tasked with keeping alive vulnerable and at-risk babies and children, and the ways in which this task is doomed in a society that can't bear to really know about our violence towards children (and in this respect his critique echoes Coe's chapter discussing similar dynamics in relation to professional boundary violations). He analyses the vilification of social workers in the Cleveland Inquiry, where children believed to have been sexually abused were removed from their families; and he describes this as a kind of social repression *barrier that gives rise to the relentless assaults on the profession of social work in the context of high profile cases of child fatalities. As Neeld and Clarke did in their opening chapter, describing the work with mothers and babies referred by social services for assessment, so too here, Cooper begins his account at 'the scene of the crime' – in this case, the moment when the state turned upon its own agents of statutory regulation and scapegoated social workers for the unbearable, unknowable societal violence represented by the 'Baby P' case.*

INTRODUCTION

This chapter centres on a particular story, which is told as a kind of post-modern crime thriller. I follow in the footsteps of one well-known example of the thriller genre which reveals the identity of the villain and shows the scene of the crime at the beginning. For readers old enough to remember the original series this is how every episode of *Columbo* starts, after which we sit back and watch Peter Falk artfully stumble his way towards nailing his man, or woman, as they twist and turn in the wind to evade the outcome we know to be inevitable.

This story positions the protagonist as a classically tragic victim of forces beyond his own comprehension or control. There is another narrative that would render him a more knowing and rational subject, a bit part player in the wider drama of social policy in this country over the last 15 years, twisting in different winds – of accountability discourses, political populism, and the idealisations of managerialist politics. These narratives converge in the here and now of 2011, when, after a year of Coalition government in Britain, the future of social work seems more open in certain respects, but still shaped by the dominant public narratives of the recent past – the episodic eruption of child abuse 'scandals'. How the reforms proposed in Eileen Munro's review of child protection work (2010a, b, 2011) will actually impact on policy practice remains to be decided at the time of writing, although her review is a courageous and hopeful intervention.

THE SCENE OF THE CRIME

The crime scene to which I refer was a news conference in early December 2008 at the height of the 'Baby P' crisis, when Ed Balls, Secretary of State for Children, Schools and Families, announced his decision to employ special powers to intervene and sack Sharon Shoesmith, the Director of Children's Services in Haringey, where Peter Connelly had lived and died. It took place against the backdrop of the *Sun* newspaper's petition campaign calling for the sacking of all the social workers involved in the case, naming and picturing four of them, including Sharon Shoesmith. 'And I further demand that Beverley Hughes, the Children's Minister, and Ed Balls should apply immediate and sustained pressure to ensure this happens,' the petition reads. Tabloid media pressure in this period was intense, but reached a notorious height with this front-page headline: 'Blood on Their Hands'. The hands, of course, belong not to the killers of baby Peter Connelly, but to social workers, although the lingering ambiguity is significant.

Out of the media chorus in attendance at the conference, steps a *Sun* reporter, who asks Mr Balls whether the newspaper's million signature campaign has influenced his decision to step in and sack Ms Shoesmith. In the later words of Labour back-bencher Bob Marshall-Andrews, the reporter:

no doubt on the instructions of his Editor attempted in a question to glean some credit for the *Sun* newspaper. It was a despicable thing to do and I am very sorry that my Minister Mr Balls did not have the courage in these circumstances to treat that question with the contempt that it deserved. (Marshall-Andrews 2008)

My own recollection on seeing the press conference live, which produced a kind of lurch in my guts, was that Mr Balls went slightly further, not only refusing to deny any credit to the *Sun* for his decision, but giving some grounds to suppose that he had been positively influenced in his decision by the petition campaign.

The public exposure of News International's involvement in 'communications interception' (phone hacking to most of us) in 2011 has further clarified the context of Ed Balls's lapse. It was already clear that we were witnessing a drama about public bullying. Sections of the media were bullying social workers and Haringey council; and Mr Balls, identifying with the bullies, turned on Haringey and its director of Children's Services, Sharon Shoesmith, in particular. Her employers then did little to protect her. Now it seems that successive governments and their Prime Ministers had, over decades, been almost entirely subservient to the demands and intrusions of News International. No one stood up to them for fear of being harassed, vilified, smeared.

One question facing us is this: is the bully any less individually accountable or responsible for his actions when it transpires he is in some sense the victim of, or at least a willing participant in, a generalised culture of bullying?

Opening my case for the prosecution, as it were, I want to propose that for the profession of social work this was the defining moment of the Baby Peter crisis. The events of those weeks have reverberated ever since and will do so for years to come – the pessimist in me says until the next time a similar child death is propelled into awareness in the public sphere. A number of frantic conversations from that time are lodged in my memory. One of them was with a colleague and friend working inside the Department for Children, Schools and Families who reported that the department was in a state of massive confusion, and that crazy ideas were being considered, such as privatising the whole child protection system; crazy but in a curious way also logical under the circumstances.

THE INTEGRITY OF OFFICE

In line with the 'tragic' thesis I am developing, Ed Balls' moment of identification with the mob atmosphere was an over-determined event: a moment of personal weakness perhaps, a moment of political weakness certainly, but more significantly a moment when his carriage of the integrity of public office collapsed. If the state and its offices, embodied in the figure of the Secretary of State, cannot hold its lines at the point of maximum pressure, its functionaries might be forgiven for panicking and considering the line of least resistance – expulsion of this troublesome business out of its own domain into the private sector.

The notion of public 'office' is rather unfashionable, made more so by the studied 'informality' of governmental style made popular by Tony Blair during his Prime Ministerial years: 'sofa government', as it became known, a development that returned to haunt him in very precise ways as the various Iraq war inquiries unfolded – so many crucial meetings, it emerged, at which no minutes or records of decisions were kept (Evans 2010). But in circumstances of conflict in particular, the boundaries of the offices of state are crucial frontiers between the legitimacy of the state and its democratic electoral mandate on the one hand, and the power of any pressure group, interest group, stakeholder, or mob to determine the course of public affairs on the other. We saw similar pressures bearing down upon Jack Straw during the eruption in 2010 of demands to expose the identity of Jamie Bulger's killers, a dilemma between the boundaries of justice and the impulse for vengeance. He in the end handled this rather better than Mr Balls and didn't divulge their names. Possibly, then, even governments sometimes learn from experience.

STEPS ONE, TWO...

Both situations are about the handling or mishandling of conflict. The process of government is centrally about the management of conflict. So also, I want to propose, are the primary tasks of the social work profession. However, intelligent analytical support for, or commentary on, this notion is rather rare in the social work literature. The best articulation I know of is in a very good book first published 20 years ago – *Making Sense of Social Work* by Michael Preston Shoot and Dick Agass (1990). But the book lacks attention to how this proposition translates into everyday practice experience, and this modified its influence:

From a macro to an individual micro perspective the world in which we live is riven with conflicts, divisions and tensions. It is unpredictable, uncertain and fundamentally unsafe… A struggle for power and domination characterises much human interaction. (Preston Shoot and Agass 1990, p.105)

This is step one in how to murder a profession. Invent a profession whose primary task could be described as ridding society of the burden of too much everyday awareness of its own inevitable afflictions; a profession with a special remit to intervene in the most private of spheres wherein this struggle for domination and power is not supposed to exist – the family, our haven in a heartless world.

Step two is more subtle. Do nothing to discourage the understandable zeal of many who join this profession, by promoting a fundamental category mistake. Those who join may believe that their role is not simply to protect the rest of society from too much *awareness* of these depressing realities, but to comprehensively *rid* our world of them. More modest and realistic ambitions – to undertake to make some difference to the lives of some of the most vulnerable, unwell and disadvantaged – become despised as reformist, accommodating, individualist, and psychologising. As the fantasy project of social purification gains credence within a significant sector of the workforce, and becomes hitched to wider Utopian political movements and ideologies, an enemy appears within its own professional ranks – psychoanalytic caseworkers and indeed any methodological tendencies that support sustained face-to-face work aimed at ameliorating distress and helping people recover personal agency. These gloomy individualistic realists must be expunged.

And so, in the troubled history of social work in the 20th century, they were expunged. When I entered the profession in the late 1970s, I found a civil war in progress between 'radical social work' and 'psychoanalytic casework'. Psychoanalytic casework never stood a chance in this straw man skirmish, and with its evisceration went some of the vital organs of social work's identity – the central place of proper worked-out practice methodologies for how to help real people in circumstances of actual distress. A vacuum appeared at the heart of social work's identity that has never been meaningfully filled.

We tried filling it with brave statements about 'values', but in the absence of any confident sense of *how* to actually 'empower' conflicted, damaged and often damaging people, families and communities, this was wafer-thin stuff. And I think the whole world knew it and could see it.

Of course, much good, thoughtful, robust, engaged social work practice survived, and still does. But wider society, and especially certain predatory political and media industry elements, sensed that this profession, with its weakened core identity and its thin, false-self-like veneer of defences against its own emptiness, was now ripe and ready for what was about to become its primary social function – a site for projection.

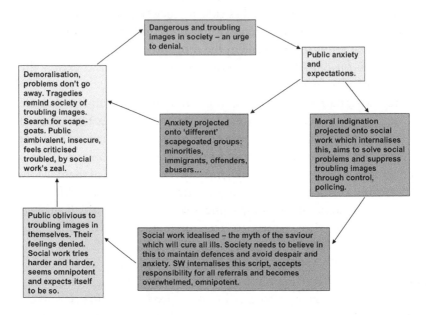

Figure 9.1 A downward spiral – outside in…inside out (adapted from Preston Shoot and Agass 1990)

This diagram, adapted from Preston Shoot and Agass's book, captures well the spirals of self-reinforcing systemic projective processes of which social work is both victim and perpetrator. But it does not explain how *this* particular profession came to be burdened in this way. Other professions, like the law, the police service, and to some degree medicine, are also centrally occupied with social conflict. Somehow, though, they manage this from within a stronger, better protected base, with clearer institutional boundaries. Situated at the crossroads of so many conflicting social currents, social work is singled out by its manifest lack of genuine *fight*, preferring as some have argued a disposition for 'fight-flight' dynamics. We have trouble standing up for ourselves, defining our aims, purposes, and the means by which we achieve these. We have rarely excited figures of political or cultural influence to champion social work (although a surprising number of ministers of state and MPs have been social workers in their time). For the same reasons, the profession has been prone to internalising, or at least failing to refuse, successive efforts at massive and violent projection into its collective psyche.

As I wrote this, I saw as if for the first time the outlines of the deeper, murkier thesis I am propounding. Ironically, in his moment of weakness, perhaps Ed Balls was behaving rather *like* a social worker, invaded by the hating certainties of the angry vengeful mob, unable to defend the integrity of his professional office, in the grip of the projections that invade a momentarily weakened identity. One could, then, connote this moment as one of projective identification – the invasion into him of a singularly potent, but most importantly *unsymbolised*, set of social anxieties and conflicts, giving rise to an excessively frightened and punitive state of mind.

But if so, what exactly are these anxieties, beyond the rather obvious coercive force exerted by any mob state of mind? This is the real mystery, and there is a mystery within the mystery. If there is a congruence between what Ed Balls found himself subjected to in that period, and what social work itself 'carries' on behalf of society the rest of the time, what does this consist of?

The history of child maltreatment and child protection in Britain over the last 30–40 years seems, from one standpoint, one of repeated and continually unresolved crisis, of which Baby Peter was just the latest manifestation. But this is not the whole story by a long way. The broader cultural narrative is indeed marked by episodic eruptions of massive and turbulent public, professional and political contestation. But a fuller historical view shows that some of the acute contests of the last 30 years have in fact resulted in clear 'settlements' representing solid and impressive achievements in our social capacity to tolerate and engage with the realities of child maltreatment, while others have not.

I will review this history as succinctly as possible – taking in the Cleveland crisis of 1987, the associated eruption of Satanic Abuse allegations, and of course the successive eruptions of public concern over the deaths of children known to, or in the care of, services.

STEP THREE…

But this dual perspective – of genuine achievement masked by the cloak of so-called failure – discloses a third crucial step in how to prepare the ground for a murder. Social work has become steadily, insidiously identified in the public mind, with its alleged 'failures'. Its public 'failures' have been in the realm of child protection. Social work has become identified with child protection work; and finally child protection work has become equivalent to social work, despite repeated efforts to establish the reality of the former as a 'multi-agency' responsibility. In one language this represents a breakdown in 'asymmetrical' thinking in favour of symmetrical part-whole equivalences; in another language it can of course be construed as 'part object' relating by the wider society towards one of its own sub-systems. But whatever, it creates a psychosocial context in which no other profession much wants to assume the responsibilities with which social work is saddled, and speculatively also, a situation in which a beleaguered Secretary of State might unconsciously think that a choice about whether to side with social work or the will of the mob was something of a 'no brainer'.

A HISTORICAL CORRECTIVE: THE TWO TASKS OF THE CHILD PROTECTION SYSTEM

Now, how did this state of affairs arise? In truth, neither child protection work nor social work in this country has been a failure. But both have somehow ended up in a profoundly beleaguered condition, largely imprisoned by the defensive proceduralised and electronic systems of control which have arisen largely in response to the successive moral panics about child maltreatment that I alluded to. This development cannot really be understood without attention to the dual primary task of the child protection system in society that I have hinted at.

In summary I suggest that the child protection system as a whole has two primary tasks: an explicit or overt one of acting to protect the most vulnerable children from serous harm – a task at which, on some indices at least, it does quite well. Its second, implicit or perhaps unconscious, primary task is to protect the wider society from dangerous and disturbing knowledge. To put it slightly differently, this second primary task is to manage on behalf of the rest of adult society our deep ambivalence about children, about parenting, and about the propensity in all of us to feel like doing violence towards our own children; in other words the ubiquity of ordinary hatred within the everyday job of parenting.

Viewed like this, the system functions in Wilfred Bion's terms as a 'specialised work group' on behalf of society (Bion 1961). This might be an appealing idea within the psychoanalytic community, but it is a difficult proposition for which to find real evidence. Here I offer just one or two morsels starting with a few lines from the novelist Rachel Cusk's uncomfortably honest book about her experience of motherhood:

> Looking after children is a low status occupation. It is isolating, frequently boring, relentlessly demanding and exhausting. It erodes your self-esteem and your membership of the adult world. The more it is separated from the rest of life, the harder it gets... As a mother you learn what it is to be both martyr and devil. In motherhood I have experienced myself as both more virtuous and more terrible, and more implicated too in the world's virtue and terror, than I would from the anonymity of childlessness have thought possible. (Cusk 2002, pp.7–8)

However, for a significant proportion of the population, official or media recognition of child maltreatment will not be functioning as a vehicle to assuage conscious or unconscious anxieties (it's OK, the real abusers are over there and being dealt with by those social workers), but as a representation of realities known to them, but not publicly disclosed or investigated. How come?

Child maltreatment remains a major public health and social-welfare problem in high-income countries. Every year, about 4–16 per cent of children are physically abused and one in ten is neglected or psychologically abused. During childhood, between 5 per cent and 10 per cent of girls and up to 5 per cent of boys are exposed to penetrative sexual abuse, and up to three times this number are exposed to any type of sexual abuse. However, official rates for substantiated child maltreatment indicate less than a tenth of this burden (Gilbert *et al.* 2008).

So, up to ten times the amount of child abuse ever reported or investigated in this country is lurking somewhere just beneath public, judicial, community or professional awareness. We might then wonder, what is the contribution of this 'hidden' population of abusing and abused adults and young people to eruptions of public outrage and anxiety, when a child abuse case hits the headlines?

TRUTH, KNOWLEDGE AND FANTASY: A SOCIAL DIALOGUE ABOUT CHILD ABUSE

I want to suggest that each time that wider society is confronted with new awareness of something like the *actual* prevalence of abuse in its midst, the impact of this new knowledge is traumatic, in some meaningful sense of that rather abused word. Of course the truly traumatic events – such as the widespread intra-familial sexual abuse of children – have already occurred; but our collective capacity to tolerate knowing about this may not be securely established, so much so that under some circumstances there may not even be a language, an available conceptual apparatus or discourse with which individuals or society can think about such matters. A kind of social repression barrier is operating (see also Chapters 7 and 10).

In Figure 9.2, I represent what I see as certain very turbulent, but ultimately positive processes in which the specialised professional system of child protection was pressed into a complex philosophical dialogue with the remainder of society. The Cleveland crisis of 1987, in which over two hundred children from a single local authority were taken into care on grounds of suspected intra-familial sexual abuse in the space of a few weeks, is the first example. With Cleveland there really was a world before and a world after. In the course of a few turbulent months, as the extraordinary events in Cleveland unfolded, our world changed, and changed I believe decisively for the better. The fact of widespread intra-familial sexual abuse in our society became established, accepted where previously it was almost completely denied or unrecognised. But not without a tremendous struggle; it is easy to forget how ill-equipped we were at that time as a society and as individuals to cope with the emergence into social awareness of this most disturbing of social facts. In retrospect it can seem as though a capacity to tolerate painful and unwelcome truths won out in a contest with the impulse to deny them, and to label the truth-seekers mad. While this is accurate, and this was a crisis in which an opportunity for civilised progress was seized, it seems we forget that, at the time, most of us were truly uncertain about the status of the disclosures and revelations which were emerging. Sexual abuse as a widespread social reality was breaking through a social repression barrier. However, Cleveland became a social 'crisis' not just because new and disturbing facts were emerging into the daylight, but also because these 'facts' sometimes transpired to be *inherently* uncertain in their nature, independently of any social, political, ideological or organisational pressure brought to bear by interested parties in the context of their emergence.

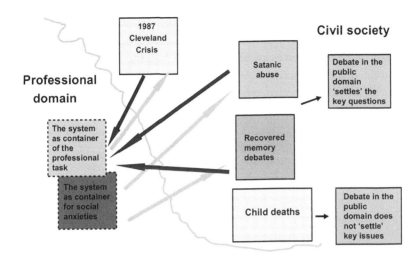

Figure 9.2 The two dimensions of child protection work as a process of achieving social 'settlement': 'What is true? What should we believe? What kinds of abuse exist, or not?'

In certain circumstances in sexual abuse, no-one, not even the victim, may be entirely sure 'what happened'. This fact – the fact of inherent indeterminacy or undecidability with respect to historical truths about abuse – seems to me to be an important but under-recognised component in the construction of the crisis. It may be true, as Freud (1950) claimed, that the incest taboo is the foundation stone of civilisation, securing the boundary between reality-based and fantasy-based social and psychological functioning, but it then follows that where this boundary has been violated, something fundamental about our grip on the epistemological foundations of civilisation will be compromised. This is a pretty frightening discovery. However, after a period of testing in the public domain, in the courts and the inquiry process itself, something like a 'true' overall position was settled upon – the ordinary prevalence of widespread intra-familial abuse was accepted as a reality. There has been no subsequent publicly endorsed effort to overturn this 'settlement'.

The second episode concerns what became known as 'Satanic abuse'. This, as some may recall, was one dimension of the Orkneys crisis, but there were other sites of alleged exposure of Satanic abuse – especially in Rochdale and Nottingham. If the fact, the existence or otherwise, of child sexual abuse was temporarily and fiercely contested during the Cleveland affair, then the Satanic abuse disclosures led to even more controversial contestations. Broadly, and I suspect correctly, the weight of official evidence and opinion eventually settled on a judgement that the most extreme features of allegations of Satanic abuse were a kind of hysteria or group fantasy. Along the way, some careful distinctions were established: the evidence for ritual abuse, and systems of organised child abuse, became better accepted and understood, but the more lurid allegations associated with Satanic abuse – sacrificial baby murder, cannibalism, drinking the blood of murdered children – were rejected. In thorough international studies not a single shred of forensic evidence was discovered to support these claims.

To give us a flavour of where the controversy came to rest, here is one of the conclusions of Jean La Fontaine's research study, commissioned by government to try to investigate the allegations and settle the debate:

> Rites that allegedly include the torture and sexual abuse of children and adults, forced abortion and human sacrifice, cannibalism and bestiality may be labelled satanic or Satanist. *Their defining characteristic is that the sexual and physical abuse of children is part of rites directed to a magical or religious objective. There is no evidence that these have taken place in any of the 84 cases studied.* (La Fontaine 1994, p.30; original emphasis)

The emergent claims in relation to both child sexual abuse and Satanic abuse were projected across the boundary of the professional practice system, beyond the remit of local judicial procedure or media debate, and were then subject to processes of very public national media, legal and research scrutiny. Both the Cleveland Inquiry itself, chaired by Justice Butler-Sloss, and Jean la Fontaine were obliged to engage with some deep philosophical issues to which I have alluded – what kind of thing actually 'exists' or is 'happening' in this area and how secure are our knowledge claims in relation to these phenomena – questions that philosophers would call 'ontological' and 'epistemological' respectively. To establish and create social acceptance of new and disturbing social facts of this kind, and to arbitrate conclusively on the status of some closely related social fantasies, are considerable social achievements – assuming the correct judgements were reached.

By contrast with the episodes I have just reviewed, in which accusations of incompetence, failure, and ideological zeal also abounded, what marks out the eruptions of anxiety in relation to child deaths is their refusal to, as it were, be laid to rest. There is no sign of any 'closure' around this. And what receives less attention here is the idea that these crises may be more directly associated with our response to children themselves, and the deaths of particular children, than their terrible suffering at the hands of adults of which we learn.

There are different points at which this familiar narrative could be said to begin. I take the series of child deaths in the 1980s that became the subject of high profile public inquiries as a point of departure – Jasmine Beckford, Kimberley Carlyle, Tyra Henry. Everywhere, in the wake of each of these inquiries, procedures were tightening, volumes of new guidance and procedure being written, risk assessment protocols drafted. Such was the dominant policy response, one with which we are now so familiar that it is hard to imagine it could be different.

The story continues through the 1990s and into our own decade with periods of relative calm and re-grouping, when the work of child safeguarding professionals is mostly beneath the social radar, punctuated by occasional dramatic explosions. Each time one of these occurs, government reacts to public outrage and panic by constructing a further set of rigid procedural or quasi-judicial defences, and projecting them back into the professional system, where they are at best ambivalently received, but never openly challenged. To a psychotherapist, they appear to be obsessional defences – a lot of ritual checking and re-checking, with an increasing uncertainty about what we are checking *for*. Like all dysfunctional defensive systems, they work up to a point, but they also definitely don't. Whatever is dammed up behind them keeps breaking through.

So, what is it about these admittedly dreadful and painful child murders that keeps them 'alive' as a source of public anxiety and media outrage that is continually projected back into the profession of social work?

MOURNING AND ITS RELATIONSHIP TO CHILD DEATH

It was during the Victoria Climbié inquiry that it first occurred to me that the inquiry itself, culminating in the publication of the report, might constitute an unrecognised process of public mourning. To me it is striking how in every public inquiry process and accompanying media storm, the ordinary emotional registration of the death of the child is lost, or obscured behind the intense preoccupation with questions of blame, accountability, retribution, reconstruction of missed opportunities and so on. And yet, over the last three decades, the names of perhaps half a dozen of these same children have become inscribed in public memory and discourse, and the (to coin a phrase) often monumentally long and weighty reports of the inquiry into their deaths sit in every academic and many public libraries. Beyond, somewhere out of public reach, are the memories of all the others who died similar deaths, but attained no such collective recognition. Like the tomb of the unknown soldier, does each of these inquiries and reports become the one that stands for the many?

In his book *The New Black: Mourning, Melancholia and Depression* Darian Leader (2008) devotes much interesting space to the relationship between public and private mourning. I take this quote as just one of many possible useful points of departure:

> Most Western human beings in fact watch images of death every night in the TV shows about crime scene investigation and murder that fill up the evening programme schedule. It is amazing to realize that this is what most people do after work: they watch programmes in which someone dies and whose death is subsequently explained and made sense of. The fact that this is reiterated endlessly suggests that death is ultimately not something that can be made sense of. And that the increasingly violent images multiply in the absence of a symbolic framework that might mediate them. (Leader 2008, p.74)

Do we possess a public symbolic framework to make sense of, mediate, child murder and torture in our society? I suspect not. Earlier I suggested that each eruption of new awareness in relation to child (sexual) abuse was succeeded by a process in which public institutions were engaged in an effort at some sort of 'sense making', and that the evidence is that these may have been broadly successful. The wearisome and professionally damaging repetition of eruptions over several decades with respect to child deaths suggests something different, but what? Darian Leader takes an observation of Melanie Klein's about internal processes of mourning as the departure point for his discussion of the private-public relationship that he calls 'a dialogue of mournings'.

In the mourner's state of mind, the feelings of his internal objects are also sorrowful. In his mind they share his grief in the same way as actual kind parents would. The poet tells us that 'Nature mourns with the mourner' (Klein 1975, p.359).

Contemporary controversies over the phenomenon of public mourning are telling here, says Leader. Critics of, say, the outbreak of public mourning at the death of Diana Princess of Wales who characterised the public demonstrations of grief as cynical or inauthentic are missing the point. No-one really could seriously argue that these tears are (only) for the dead figure themselves. 'Rather,' he says, 'it is the public framework that allows people to articulate their own grief for other, unrelated losses… This is a basic function of public mourning rituals. The public facilitates the private' (2008, p.77). On this argument we could recognise the now widespread public practice of establishing temporary shrines at the site of a death or loss – road accidents for example – usually in the form of collections of flowers, as an effort to establish or re-establish a wider public symbolic framework for mourning than private burial rites allow.

Darian Leader explores the many vicissitudes of the mourning process both intra-psychically, and socially, via the anthropology of mourning rituals in various societies. In some societies these rites entail a concrete re-ordering of social relationships in the community. 'After mourning and burial rites, social structures change, and formal rules govern the new set of ancestors to their descendants. The key is that the dead are installed in the ancestral line' (2008, p.116). To achieve this, he argues that the dead must be killed a second time. '(F)or the living to feel safe and secure, the dead have to die twice. Real biological death is thus different from proper symbolic death' (2008, p.116).

We might think here both of the impulsive and reactive re-ordering of professional systems that usually follows inquiries, and of the inevitability, as we put it, that 'heads will roll' somewhere in those same systems. Only then, at a public level, can the symbolic death be secured – and this I suggest is the drama in which Ed Balls became destined to enact his part.

THE TRAGIC CONCLUSION

The core thesis I have been outlining is that the social history of child abuse in Britain is about a gradual and episodic struggle to accommodate new and disturbing knowledge of ourselves, and along the way to better delineate reason from unreason. It involves a rather Hegelian idea of social science as the unfolding of society's consciousness of itself. But if, as Leader suggests, we cannot ultimately make sense of actual death, are we condemned forever to repeat the history of our knowledge of child torture and death in the manner of Jasmine Beckford, Victoria Climbié and Peter Connelly?

I am talking here about ghosts. But not the friendly sort who appear at the top of the stairs for a moment, or rattle a few jars in the kitchen.

These are the angry, vengeful, ghosts of classical tragedy who pursue their murderers or haunt those who must mourn the dead. They are the manifestation of our unfinished psychic business. They announce to us the guilt we must bear but cannot, and the loss whose recognition might send us mad. Who are the millions of people, whom I have perhaps thoughtlessly named a mob, who signed the *Sun* petition? What is propelling them to such extremes? What is in their minds? It's hard to really know, and I have come across only one serious attempt to research such a question. The characters peopling their drama are to some extent legible – the dreadfully suffering, tortured, dead infant or toddler; the evil, dangerous murderer; the complicit bystander who welcomes the murderer into the home for her own sexual gratification; and of course the abysmally incompetent and failed rescuers.

In his short book about tragedy, Adrian Poole says:

> Ghosts – Tragedy is full of them…(they) bear down on the nearest and dearest who have killed them, or those who must mourn and avenge them. But there is a more political aspect to the living dead. They also bear heavily on a whole city, people, community or culture, in so far as they embody values, ideas, and ethics that challenge the present and obstruct the future. (Poole 2005, pp.33–35)

So, my more sympathetic prosecution case against Mr Balls ends something like this (but there is another case in which he is straightforwardly charged with dereliction of public duty). Lurking beneath the official statistics on child abuse and child deaths, behind the scenes of the besieged social services offices, under the surface of the voluminous policy guidance, is a vast underworld of half-mourned or unmourned and damaged children, mostly living on inside the minds of grown adults; and a vast underworld of guilt-stricken parents who must live every day with the real or fantasised reproaches of their children, living and dead. Adrian Poole quotes a comment on another recent tragedy – the Chinese cockle-pickers of Morecombe Bay – 'It takes a tragedy to open a sudden, surprising window.'

In the case of Baby Peter this window was, in some true sense, opened by the actions or inaction of a number of social workers, doctors, and others working in desperately unfavourable organisational conditions created in part by the earlier tragedy of Victoria Climbié. Faced with that *Sun* reporter, I think Mr Balls sensed not just an angry mob who might lynch him if he did not throw them a sacrificial victim, but also the presence of a spectral army, a horde of vengeful ghosts seeking justice.

If so, he might be forgiven for metaphorically raising his dagger, and plunging it into the fragile and disparaged heart of those who opened the window admitting them into public awareness.

During every eruption of acute public anxiety about murder, violence or sexuality – but most of all when all three are involved – it becomes impossible to think straight, such is the primitive potency of the anxieties unleashed. But it remains our responsibility to try to forge understanding retrospectively, in the hope that we can prevent history of this kind repeating itself. This chapter is a contribution to that effort.

REFERENCES

Bion, W.R. (1961) *Experiences in Groups*. London: Tavistock.

Cusk, R. (2002) *A Life's Work: On Becoming a Mother*. London: Fourth Estate.

Evans, J. (2010) 'The Psychology of Spin.' Unpublished Tavistock Policy Seminar paper, 11 February 2010.

Freud, S. (1950) *Totem and Taboo*. London: Routledge and Kegan Paul.

Gilbert, R. *et al.* (2008) 'Burden and consequences of child maltreatment in high income countries.' *The Lancet*. Published online DOI: 10.1016/S0140-6736(08)61706-7.

Klein, M. (1975) 'A contribution to the psychogenesis of manic-depressive states.' In *Love, Guilt and Reparation*. London: Hogarth. (First published 1935.)

La Fontaine, J. (1994) *The Extent and Nature of Organised and Ritual Abuse: Research Findings*. London: HMSO.

Leader, D. (2008) *The New Black: Mourning, Melancholia and Depression*. London: Penguin.

Marshall-Andrews, R. (2008) 'Any Questions?' BBC Radio 4, 5 December 2008.

The Munro Review of Child Protection Part 1: A Systems Analysis (2010a) London: The Stationery Office.

The Munro Review of Child Protection, Interim Report: The Child's Journey (2010b) London: The Stationery Office.

The Munro Review of Child Protection, Final Report: A Child Centred System (2011) London: The Stationery Office.

Poole, A. (2005) *Tragedy: A Very Short Introduction*. Oxford: Oxford University Press.

Preston Shoot, M. and Agass, D. (1990) *Making Sense of Social Work: Psychodynamics and Systems in Practice*. London: MacMillan.

Chapter 10

COUPLES WHO KILL
The Malignant Bonding

Estela Welldon

In this chapter Estela Welldon discusses how and why couples kill, exploring notorious cases in the public domain. As with the preceding chapter by Cooper, so too here the 'milieu' is the public domain itself, and the (idealized) private family unit taken to be at its centre. She demonstrates how toxic dynamics within couples, which she terms 'malignant bonding', create situations where children are killed. These parents themselves destroy the private milieu of the family. When this violence is discovered and the hidden world of the family is brutally exposed to the public there is a passionate outcry from all sides, disavowing all knowledge of such brutality. Welldon describes how the inner world of the family can be a violent and hidden space, terribly idealized, its evils overlooked. She describes the development of perverse sado-masochistic relationships within couples, including the infamous case of Myra Hindley and Ian Brady, and she elucidates the terrible ways in which children can become part of the destructive excitement of the couple, resulting in their torture and death. Despite clear evidence that parents inflict harm to their offspring, the societal response to intrafamilial violence continues to be denial, horror and disbelief.

INTRODUCTION
In this chapter I shall concentrate on the dynamic description of a horrific, disturbing and somewhat unexpected phenomenon that I have termed 'malignant bonding'. Just by listening to patients with an open and unprejudicial mind I have come across and been able to learn of unsuspected predicaments previously unrecognized. This has, unwittingly, placed me in the role of the 'messenger' of 'bad', 'horrid news'.

My clinical research into women mistreating children, their own or others, was published in 1988 in my book *Mother, Madonna, Whore:*

The Idealization and Denigration of Motherhood. It concerns the 'awful' situations which can occur in the most sacred bonding, namely, between mother and child.

Earlier on it had been assumed that perversions were the exclusive domain of men because they were organized around the penis. To some of my male colleagues this meant that, since women didn't have penises, they couldn't have perversions – and this thought challenged me. It made me think of Freud's aphorism that the Oedipus complex in girls is resolved when they are able to have a phantasy about Daddy's babies inside, so for the first time, babies and penises were equated. My own view is that women in perversions act against their own bodies, or at least what they consider to be extensions of themselves – their babies.

For the first time the conceptualization of female perversion was made in which some very emotionally damaged women were using motherhood as a vehicle for their perversion. As such, I noticed that some women were acting in harmful physical and/or sexual ways against themselves, or against their children. In these cases, babies were experienced as extensions of themselves.

Ethel Person (1994), in a rich and comprehensive study of the beating and sado-masochistic fantasies in women, coined both terms 'the body silenced' (meaning the lack of sexual desire) and 'the body as the enemy' (meaning hypochondriac symptoms). I believe that a fitting term for my female patients' specific predicaments in relation to their bodies and babies could be 'the body as the torturer'. This would signal the compulsive urges these women experience towards their bodies, unconsciously making them function as the effective torture tool in their becoming victimizers to themselves and to their babies. There are also present different degrees of disassociation, the most severe corresponding to Munchausen's syndrome by proxy. At other times, such as entering into sado-masochistic relationships, the partner is unconsciously designated as the torturer.

Later on, again, guided by my clinical experience, I was able to observe sado-masochistic patterns in couples, which were usually the result of being subjected from very early on to neglect and abuse. But, as painful as the work is, it is also possible to find rich rewards. For example, now, 23 years since *Mother, Madonna, Whore* was published, neglect and abuse within the family is widely recognized and many preventative measures have been taken to avoid the expansion and escalation of such bizarre actions.

In 2005, there was a TV dramatization of the case of Beverly Allit, the nurse who in the course of her duties killed several children. We were able to hear comments, including feelings of guilt, by some of her colleagues, who, at the time, were blissfully unaware of the proximity of a serial killer, mainly because she was a woman – demonstrating a 'prejudice' against the idea of a woman as a serial killer, let alone of children!

The problem of prejudices is that we close our minds to anything that could be 'undesirable' or 'ugly' but simultaneously we are aware that people feel titillated by the most salacious details about individuals who commit all sorts of crimes, especially sexual ones. This is obviously created by intellectual laziness accompanied by the associated feeling of being virtuous in comparison to people who do these 'horrid' things. I think that as a 'caring society' we should all feel at least partly responsible for the lack of concern and awareness of horrors that happen next door. Again and again neighbours only seem able to talk after the terrible deeds have been exposed, including the case of the West family and more recently the Garrido couple in California and others.

There are several examples from the media and history in which the female partner's actions and participation have been blatantly obvious, for example Myra Hindley and Rosemary West. There are others, such as Nancy Garrido, wife of Phillip, who appears to be forever a victim of her husband's sadistic and crazy behaviour. However, she was in active collusion in the abduction of Jaycee Duggard and for the next 19 years a silent witness of his physical rape and sexual abuse of the young captive girl and his fathering of her two daughters. Also later on she was an active participator in sexually molesting and harassing other young girls under her husband's guidance. Jaycee Duggard (2011) wrote *A Stolen Life*, which is her account of her experiences.

Other women's participation is not so obviously in the open, their cruelty, collusion and engagement only apparent by their inaction, silence and 'ignorance' in the presence of all sorts of 'eccentric', 'mad' behaviour of their husbands, for example the case of Rosemarie Fritzl, wife of the notorious Joseph. The UK has its own version of the Austrian case in the 'Sheffield incest case' in which a mother disappeared, unable to tolerate her husband's cruelty but leaving their two daughters available for the father's sexual abuse, reflected in the repeated rape and fathering of children.

At this juncture I shall describe the interactions between partners and the harmful actions against children produced by both together.

Strange as it may seem, child abuse can be initiated, and even stimulated, not only by the man but also by the woman in the couple. We are no longer talking of who is the victim or perpetrator within the couple: they are partners with equal participation in the design and execution of their actions in response to their own severe very early traumatic experiences. In fact, the difference between male and female perverse actions, as earlier asserted, lies in the 'location' of the object or target: whereas in men it is usually directed towards the outside, in women it is either against themselves, against their bodies in self-destructive patterns, or against objects of their own creations – that is, their babies.

There are two famous and notorious cases in England of 'malignant bonding' – one, Myra Hindley and Ian Brady, with an extra-familial configuration, whilst the other, Fred and Rosemary West, is within a family – and they come to my mind when thinking of the interactions between both partners and their harmful actions produced by both together against children, their own and others.

Pursuing my own findings, I would like to emphasize the strong reaction of disbelief that the women in question could have had anything to do, in any active way, in the horrible actions against the children. Everyone – from lay public to all professionals, including experienced judges – tacitly assumed that, if at all involved, these two women were responding to bullying and threats from their male partners.

The first case goes back to 1964 and was dramatized and screened in October 2006 for television by Channel 4 under the name of *Longford*. Lord Longford was a very compassionate and religious, although rather naïve, eccentric aristocrat Englishman who took care of some of the most difficult and at times impossible law cases. He had a belief that he could not only understand better but also help those he saw as victims of miscarriages of justice. He was a strong believer in hope and change (and redemption), even in the most intractable cases. He became famous for his intense interest and activity surrounding Myra Hindley after she was sentenced. This is the woman who, with her partner and lover Ian Brady, abducted children, on many different occasions, in the north of England. Together, after subjecting the children to acts of torture, including sexual violence and rape, some of which they recorded, they eventually killed and buried them on the moors. Despite Lord Longford being in active service during wartime, he was stunned by the enormity of Hindley's crimes which 'made even him pause to draw breath for a moment'. At their first meeting at Holloway, she requested that he facilitate meetings with Brady, who was serving his life sentence in a men's prison.

Longford, who was initially very much against such meetings, was eventually persuaded by Hindley and agreed to do as she had requested. From then on, and for the next 35 years, Longford continued to argue her case. Such were her formidable powers of persuasion.

The crimes committed by Hindley and her lover, Ian Brady, shocked the nation and became the benchmark by which other acts of evil came to be measured. It is revealing that, while to start with Hindley was never thought to be an active party in these horrific actions, after seeing evidence of her being active the media view of her changed totally and she was then depicted by the tabloid press as 'the most hated woman in Britain'.

On 6 May 1966, Hindley and Brady were jailed for life after a 15-day trial. The killings soon became known as the 'Moors murders', and they were made even more notorious by the tape-recording played at the trial of one of their victims pleading for her life. Hindley's active involvement in the case was now unquestionable, since the young girl was directly appealing to Myra for her release. Later on, while in prison, Hindley admitted to her active influence in all crimes. In 1994, Hindley wrote that she was 'wicked and evil' and had behaved 'monstrously'. And again: 'Without me, those crimes could probably not have been committed.'

When they originally met, Brady had a minor criminal record with stretches in borstals and prison, and, while inside, he began his fixation with Hitler and the writings of the Marquis de Sade. Myra left school at 15, learned how to type and within three years went to work at a small chemical firm. There she met Brady, who was working as a stock clerk, and fell in love with him. Once they became lovers, Hindley was prepared to do anything Brady asked. At her trial, evidence was produced that she had been subjected to threats, violence, and intimidation by him. Again, prejudices were to the fore when, two days after the original trial, the judge who sentenced Hindley said: 'Though I believe Brady is wicked beyond belief without hope of redemption, I cannot feel that the same is necessarily true of Hindley once she is removed from his influence.'

No one, including Lord Longford, was emotionally capable at that time of seeing a woman – in this case, Myra Hindley – as being both the prompter and promoter of the malignant bonding with Brady. But, of course, who could suspect that a woman who has the capacity for pregnancy and bringing up babies is the one who may be the perpetrator? Why the reluctance on his part to consider this possibility? The Channel 4 programme suggests that it may be because he was already, in transferential terms, caught in the same process of malignant bonding with Myra. Interestingly enough, in the film, the person who almost succeeded in breaking up this relational perversion was his wife, Elizabeth. But Elizabeth Longford's opposition weakened over time. In December 1976, she finally agreed to accompany her husband to Holloway.

Surprising as it may seem, she and Hindley became firm friends. This may be further evidence of Myra's enormous powers of seduction and persuasion, and as such it becomes a potential ménage à trois, with Elizabeth as part of the parental couple, with her husband placing Myra as the 'sick baby', unable to wake up from the drug-induced, almost catatonic situation. In the film, different and varied possibilities of malignant bonding of a very perverse nature are shown. Hers and Brady's first – which, of course, is what excites the others, who are unconscious of the nature of this interest.

The West family represents the most famous UK case of family abuse, which includes the physical and sexual abuse, torture, and eventually killing of their own and other children (as well as adults). Such actions, sadly and most unfortunately, are not isolated and exclusive examples. And if this appears to be extreme and beyond the boundaries of what we are supposed to know and to be familiar with, let me tell you that this is not so. There are couples and families afflicted by this perverse behaviour who are at close quarters with us. Perhaps the degree of their perverse actions is not as extreme as the Wests', but it does require acknowledgement and professional expertise to deal with. Sachs (2008) states that 'parents who feel compelled to see their children tortured or dead have an extremely traumatic history themselves', which leads to 'the inevitability of further trauma, generation after generation' (p.132).

In the last few years we have read in the British newspapers about different couples who while performing their 'duties' as babysitters have physically and sexually abused children in their care. In February 2006, an incident was reported in the *Guardian* in which a couple had repeatedly raped a three-month-old baby. Not only that – they even took videos of all the rape scenes, performed by both partners, man and woman. More recently, on Friday 26 March 2010, a story appeared in the *Guardian* under the headline of 'Couple Face Life Terms for Murdering Boy in Their Care'. The boy, aged three years, had 70 injuries to his body. He had been neglected, abused, and beaten by a 19-year-old woman cousin of his mother and the woman's boyfriend, aged 25. The baby's mother felt unable to cope with the baby's demands and paid the couple for taking care of her baby.

I know these public cases are accounts of the most horrifying and sadistic events, but I want to make you aware of the possibilities that may or may not come your way, as an incipient awareness is essential in order to detect these happenings from very early on. In the history of psychoanalysis, there was a reluctance to take claims of sexual abuse as real, and instead these were considered to be phantasies. But today it is no longer possible to persevere with that position, since the reality is present in flagrant ways. All these public cases, and the ones I am familiar with, share a terrible feature: the strangled, panicky, unbearable pain experienced by the victims is being recorded. Technology has afforded the most sophisticated means to do so – from recording just the voices of those innocent children, as in the 1960s, to the making of home videos, now with digital cameras. And today different images such as these can be downloaded from the internet. There is thus a compulsive need to repeat again and again against themselves – the perpetrators – the tortures inflicted upon the innocent victims.

I find this feature a most distressing one, and I am reminded that Freud in *Beyond the Pleasure Principle* (1920) linked the destructive impulses and how this need to repeat, to represent, to double, and to supplement, results in either the perpetrator identifying with another or finding it impossible to determine which of the two she herself is. When perpetrators make and record, not only their own actions but also the confused, disturbed, painful, and frightened reactions of their victims, is this used as identification with their own childhood? Is it to do with their need to make themselves feel all-powerful and in complete control of the torture inflicted because they need this 'reassurance'? Is the listening/watching 'addiction' associated with early sexual abuse and the need to form sadomasochistic relationships in which they have the monopoly of power? The recording could also be used as a kind of home-made pornography for the couple; this would allow the sexual excitement gained in the torture of children to be re-created on future occasions, serving as a sexual trigger for masturbation and a manic defence against the black hole of depression.

Frequently the children involved are not even their own, just as happened with the cases described above, particularly the notorious case of Hindley and Brady. Not only did they torture and kill the children involved in their rampage of seducing, grooming and taking children away, but also they recorded their victim's voices of anguish, pain and suffering while they were being tortured to listen to on repeated occasions. Why this need to re-enact this barbaric, primitive, irrational behaviour? This is an extreme situation, but we also have equally or even more perverse behaviour in the case of the Wests. The West family tortured and killed some of their own children as well as others and kept the corpses within the walls of their own home. What should one make of this couple who had to use their own family to create their own intimate, close, family genocide and holocaust within their own home walls? After this indescribably awful discovery, it was most alarming to recognize the compelling element it provided others, with the gruesome and ghastly curiosity of looking at the 'forbidden'. How many people went to visit the Wests' 'home' – to see what? This reached such alarming proportions that a council decision was made to destroy this site.

But what is the extent to which a couple can let themselves go in order to elicit a sense of excitement so pervasive, so unreal but so enormously effectual to make them feel all-powerful, omnipotent, being able to create, destroy, and macerate lives? What is the extent of their feeling so empty, so vacuous, so dead, that in order to re-create a new life they had to pursue those horrific actions? And for our own interest here, what on earth drew these two individuals together? What was the chemistry/love/attraction that drew them together to start with and later on lead them to these joint, combined actions of reproduction, which in our view could be the product of a mature relationship – after all, isn't what we expect from couples when they develop and evolve in their relationships to pursue parenthood as a concrete symbolism, if this is allowed, as evidence of a healthy resolution, to have children, to grow a family – but then to torture, to abuse and finally to kill them and bury them within their own confines?

This conceptualization of 'malignant bonding' came to me during diagnostic sessions involving both parents, for the purpose of assessing their parenting abilities. At times I did these on my own but at other times the process was executed initially by a colleague and myself in separate sessions with both parents, and eventually in joint sessions. There is a lot to learn from observing, exploring, researching and making any sense of behaviour which involves domestic violence, including verbal, physical and sexual abuse, not discounting paternal, maternal and sibling incest but also being witness to such interactions. There are serious consequences arising from these different but related sorts of behaviours not only on direct family members but also on those of the following generations.

It seems to me that malignant bonding is often encountered in those parents who have never talked about their 'family secrets'; meaning having been themselves victims of sexual abuse of an incestuous nature. Actually, the repetition of the sadism involved in their actions becomes the actual remembering of what happened to them before. But now they are in the 'triumphant' position: not only is there a role reversal compared with when they were infants; they are now in complete control of the primary scene, no longer outside it but just like puppeteers in their joint effort to re-enact early painful experiences with those helpless children, who see their involvement as their own way of survival. But this is not enough to reassure that they have survived horrific physical and psychic damage to themselves. As soon as they are no longer in the concrete scenario of their sadistic but 'necessary' actions, their sense of control of the victim gradually becomes illusory and fades away. They wonder: were they in control or were they the victimized children dispossessed of all power? Thus they have to remind themselves that they had been in control. Hence the use of devices to listen and watch to once more create an illusory sense of being omnipotent in their minds, that, yes, they are now the executors.

It is fascinating, although at times very difficult, to get to know what makes a couple 'tick'. We have to observe and to explore how couples originate, how they meet and pursue their relationships in unconscious ways that may become conscious only later on, when they seem to have been consolidated, and only then the enormous conflicts emerge which have been hidden away. How many times have we all been witnesses to occurrences of incestuous actions from parents to children, a father or mother, who him/herself has been an early victim of child abuse? In the family dynamics, in which usually the father is the perpetrator, the mother/wife has been so far 'blissfully' unaware of this particular scenario; but when later on she is confronted with the harsh reality of the abuse, she has flashbacks and a memory of having been herself sexually abused as a child emerges with pervasive power from within. It is as if a magnet is operating in both partners at the moment of their initial meeting which was felt to be so bonding that it was equally irresistible and dangerous and as such very exciting. So exciting that falling in love was inevitable since the 'radar' was in full functioning and the polarizing aspects of the two was felt to be the perfect combination for a perfect coupling. But, this 'felt' sensation of 'equality', or better said 'sameness', was no longer enticing when the union became legalized and as such no longer taboo.

Of course, I am here not talking of conscious, rational behaviour. This couple, these two different persons, have felt themselves to be, from the moment of their first meeting, in almost automatic pilot mode, very close and united together but not knowing exactly why. However, this great sense of wonder starts fading away when the union is felt to be in some way 'contrived' or coercive from within. Now, the taboo element is no longer present and the sense of excitement is gone. What happens next? The pursuing of the transgressing has become the compelling element and as such the using and exploiting, including sexual abuse of children, starts. But, again, this is not straightforward because in some couples this is almost a necessary requirement for their own libidinal and narcissistic gratification which they obtain through the sexual molestation, abuse, and at times torture of their own children. There is an irrepressible need to continue succumbing to these transgressive actions because, just as with pornography, it makes them feel alive. They feel really dead inside themselves and their own way to make sure they are still alive is by exerting this enormous sense of power and control over their children.

But to what extent will a couple let themselves go, in order to elicit a sense of excitement so pervasive, so unreal but so bloodily effectual as to make them feel all-powerful, omnipotent, able to create, destroy and macerate lives? What is the extent of their feeling so empty, so vacuous, so dead, that in order to re-create a new life they had to pursue those horrific actions? My aim in exploring this severe psychopathology is to replace morbid curiosity with an interest in understanding more about the inherent complexities in this apparently unthinkable behaviour. The goal of forensic psychotherapy is to understand rather than to judge, regardless of how difficult this may be.

REFERENCES

BBC (2005) *Angel of Death: The Beverly Allit Story.* London: British Broadcasting Corporation.

Carter, H. (2010) 'Couple guilty of murdering toddler face life in prison.' *Guardian*, 26 March 2010.

Duggard, J. (2011) *A Stolen Life.* London: Simon and Schuster.

Freud, S. (1920) *Beyond the Pleasure Principle.* Standard Edition, 18.

Hooper, T. (director) (2006) *Longford.* UK: Granada/HBO for Channel 4.

Person, E. (1994) 'Corpo Ridotto al Silenzio, Corpo Nemico. Una Fantasia di Percosse.' In F. Molfino and C. Zinnardi (eds) *Sintomi Corpo Femminilatta.* Bologna: CLUEBB.

Sachs, A. (2008) *Forensic Aspects of Dissociative Identity Disorder.* London: Karnac.

Ward, D. (2006) 'Babysitter couple jailed for rape of 12-week-old girl.' *Guardian,* 11 January 2006.

Welldon, E.V. (1988) *Mother, Madonna, Whore: The Idealization and Denigration of Motherhood.* London: Karnac.

Part III

COURAGE UNDER FIRE

RESILIENCE, REFLECTION
AND REPARATION

I was angry with my friend:
I told my wrath, my wrath did end.
I was angry with my foe:
I told it not, my wrath did grow.

From *Songs of Innocence and Experience*,
William Blake (1789)

Chapter 11

INFANTICIDE AND PAEDOPHILIA AS A DEFENCE AGAINST INCEST
Work with a Man with a Severe Intellectual Disability[1]

Valerie Sinason

In this chapter Valerie Sinason provides us with clinical material from psychotherapy sessions with a learning disabled man and 'dustbin baby' whose violent sexual acting out came to be seen as representing a search for his parents. The tensions between 'micro' and 'macro' in Corbett's chapter are echoed and reinforced here as Sinason describes how the therapeutic milieu in the mind found a way to survive and therefore to help to process the raw and visceral traumatised distress of this troubled man, who is able to find words to describe his quest and his awareness of how the societal milieu has rubbished and disposed of him. Sinason evokes and explores the Biblical tale of Abraham and Isaac to foreground the theme of child sacrifice as it is played out both in sexual abuse and child murder and in the societal manifestations of murderousness towards foetuses identified as disabled.

INTRODUCTION
Working with children and adults with severe learning disabilities who have experienced institutional and/or domestic abuse throws light on the painful links between unworked-through victim experiences and the need to perpetrate. Indeed, when working with a population who have had little access to talking therapies and whose struggle to make sense of unbearable trauma is exacerbated by organic limitations and impingements (see Chapter 15), it is remarkable that there is not far more offending behaviour. With scant literature available for those with low reading ages, outside of the Books Beyond Words pioneering

---

1   An earlier version of this chapter was presented to a day workshop at the Institute of Contemporary Psychoanalysis, Los Angeles.

series, and with rare access to relevant films and plays, the usual ways in which people learn to process their developmental traumas through internalising culture are not available.

It is hard to imagine what it is like for a child or adult silenced through abuse whose intellectual disabilities make it impossible to process the trauma. Indeed, it is a hypothesis of mine that so-called autistic repetition and echolalia is misperceived and represents a literal account of trauma (Sinason 2004). At my first meeting with a woman with a severe intellectual disability, she slowly repeated the words 'uncle Ed' with increasing emphasis. On her ward they referred to her as the one who always says 'uncle-ed'. The words had lost their meaning. Her two-word life history that had frozen her hope and development had been relegated to a dissociative diagnostic term for the purpose of avoiding her pain. Until I properly could help her unpick the trauma he had caused her, she was stuck in societal denial.

Abuse is widespread as an emotional, physical, sexual and spiritual event in the lives of children and adults with intellectual disabilities (Sinason 1992, 1996, 2011), and the work of organisations such as RESPOND with Alan Corbett, Tamsin Cottis, Richard Curen, Liz Lloyd, Shanawaz Haque and the IPD (Institute for Psychotherapy and Disability) have highlighted this.

In many fields, work with abusers and victims is often split. Indeed, this can apply to the physical fabric of the building. The Tavistock and Portman Trust, for example, has separate buildings for the two groups. However, individuals and groups working with people with intellectual disability are far more aware of the meaning of being a victim-perpetrator and work, as at RESPOND, with young people and adults whose behaviour has communicated both sides of that dynamic (see Chapter 3). This means managing the clinical tension of different transference and counter-transference to both sides of the spectrum of victim-perpetratorhood within the same mind and body. It is therefore imperative to take seriously the enormity of offending behaviour at the same time as making a space for the victim.

Griffiths, Hingsburger and Christian (1985) found that the nature of deviant sexual behaviour is similar for both intellectually disabled and non-intellectually disabled offenders but the sex offender with intellectual disabilities is less likely to reach the courts and therefore treatment (Breen and Turk 1991), and his crimes are more likely to be detected. However, there is some evidence that intellectually disabled offenders can become more violent (Gilby, Wolf and Goldberg 1989) and are more likely to find male than female victims (Gilby *et al*. 1989; Griffiths *et al*. 1985). All too often, the offending is minimised with comments like, 'He is only trying to play with someone of his own developmental age,' or, the more familiar split in viewing offenders, 'He is uninhibited because of his disability and therefore more dangerous and should be removed from society.'

In this paper I want to explore severe perversion as a creative attachment-based solution to unbearable circumstances. While the solution is often inevitably socially unacceptable, illegal and destructive it is easy to overlook the co-existing courage and creativity in finding any modus vivendi. As with de Zulueta (1993) I see perversion as a consequence of childhood trauma, neglect and abuse and share Stoller's (1975) observation that 'the hostility in perversion takes form in a fantasy of revenge hidden in the actions that make up the perversion and serves to convert childhood trauma to adult triumph.'

I have the permission of Isaac to speak about him but have altered certain background details to enhance confidentiality. Isaac asked me to provide a name for him for the purpose of this chapter and I have chosen a biblical one with symbolic meaning.

BACKGROUND TO THE REFERRAL OF ISAAC BROWN

Isaac Brown (not his real name) was wringing his hands, turning them white. A 40-year-old with a severe intellectual disability, he had been referred for a risk assessment. His long-stay hospital was closing and he was going to be placed in a 'home' in the community – his first ever non-institutional base. From the moment de-institutionalisation was raised he had become interested in the idea of sexually attacking small boys and babies and spoke about this frequently.

He was found with his hands around the neck of a vulnerable visiting young child and anally masturbated publicly when children's programmes were on television. He disturbed his nurse by stating that he would either marry a little boy or kill one. At the same time, he began to make suicidal comments. Otherwise his conversation was rambled accounts of the life of Jesus and Muhammad.

It was only when he attacked a child that there was suddenly an urgent wish to seek help. Having heard his sexual, religious and suicidal ruminations from the moment he knew his hospital would close, staff were traumatised and urgent in their communications. After several phone calls and a letter, the following background could be established.

Mr Brown had a tragic history. At just a few hours old he had been found by a policeman in a dustbin in a deserted alley, wrapped in a dirty shawl. There was nothing to identify him. He was initially named after the policeman who had found him and kept his surname although he never saw him again. There were no records of his early life in which he had stayed in children's homes and hospitals that had since closed down. For the last 15 years he had been in a stable albeit unenriching environment – a vast old hospital. In this period, until news of the closure, he had been a 'trustee', one of those old-time inmates who helped staff with their duties.

The social worker said she was concerned Mr Brown would be in danger of killing himself or a child if he were not treated. She was furious with a previous psychiatric report that minimised his dangerousness where the psychiatrist had considered Mr Brown was only sexually inappropriate as a result of his severe intellectual disability: 'He is only interested in little boys because that is the level he has reached developmentally.' It was only because of that report that he had further freedom of movement within the hospital and was being considered for community care.

Indeed, this is not unusual. Those with an intellectual disability are seen not only as Children of a Lesser God (as the superb film title of that name showed) but, equally dangerously, Children of a Lesser Satan. Watching someone anally masturbate, threaten suicide and approach little children is a frightening and numbing experience – it stupefies, and as a result of such trauma there is a wish to avoid thinking and minimise the worrying observation.

This was the first time I had agreed to assess a man who had attempted to strangle a child. I was frightened. However, it was important for me to note that he had *not* strangled the child, although there was ample opportunity. With regard to the murderous wish to strangle babies I was thinking of hatred for the disabled self being projected on to 'normal' babies.

MEETING WITH MR BROWN

Mr Brown was brought to see me by two escorts. I was surprised to realise that the moment I saw him all fear left me and was replaced by an acute sympathy. This did not extend to his escorts. Both men had blank faces and were clearly not invested with any hope or interest for the event. However, when I asked them to wait outside the room one of the men came to life and raised an eyebrow and looked at me contemptuously.

Mr Brown was a short, thin, agitated man who had clearly failed to thrive in childhood. His skin colour was a faded brown but his eyes were a surprising bright blue. Not only was his parentage unknown but his racial mixture was also hard to determine. Perhaps linked to this was his regular speaking of both Muhammad and Jesus.

When he entered my consulting room I said, 'Hello, I am Valerie Sinason. You can call me Dr Sinason or Valerie – how would you like me to address you?' I have always been concerned at the importance of addressing people with intellectual disabilities properly, as too often their names are lost. Of course, in Mr Brown's case, it was even more poignant.

'Isaac. Call me Isaac. I should have been called Dustbin… Dustbin! Blue-eyed boy dustbin!' he laughed, showing his decayed teeth. 'I was found in a dustbin. Who is Isaac? I never met him. Me. I am a dustbin. I should be called Isaac Dustbin. Nothing Dustbin.'

I said his name did not feel as if it belonged to him. Without a Mum or Dad to name him and know him he felt like rubbish.

He fell silent. He was wearing dirty, ragged clothes and had apparently refused the new clean clothes staff offered him.

IB: 'Do you know your name?'

VS: 'What do you think?'

IB: 'You got a mum and dad. Like Muhammad and Jesus. You know your name.'

There was a long poignant silence. I did not speak of Muhammad or Jesus as I did not yet understand what those religious figures meant to him.

VS: 'That is really hard. You have lived for 40 years and you do not know who your parents are, what they look like and what your name would have been had they stayed to be a family with you.'

IB: 'Dead,' he whispered.

VS: 'They might be dead. If you are 40 they could be anything from their late 50s and you do not know what has happened to them.'

He looked at me intently.

IB: 'Children come from parents, like Muhammad had a father even though he died.'

VS: Yes. Even if they disappear or die it takes two people to make a baby and they are still your biological parents.'

IB: 'How old are you?'

VS: 'I wonder what you think?'

IB: 'Not my mother.'

He started wringing his hands again and rocking up and down on the chair.

IB: 'There's children in the community.'

VS: 'Yes.'

IB: 'Children are small.'

VS: 'Yes.'

IB: 'They walk by themselves. They go into shops. They visit friends. They go to school.'

VS: 'Yes. How do you feel about that?'

IB: 'Small people. Strange small people. They have mummies and daddies who don't look after them. Go to shops on their own. Stupid children. Don't take care. Go into shops by themselves or stay outside in prams or push-chairs.'

Silence.

His hands were on his penis, which was clearly erect through his tracksuit bottoms, something I used to call 'paedophile pyjamas' in my work with intellectually disabled offenders.

VS: 'If children go out without parents you think it serves them right and it serves their parents right if they are in danger.'

His eyes lit up.

IB: 'They wouldn't get hurt if at home. Can get strangled, raped, you know, willies up their bum, tied up.'

VS: 'If parents and children stayed together nothing bad would happen.'

IB: 'That's right. You're right.'

Long silence.

    VS: 'You know, you started thinking about little children just after you worked out I wasn't your mum.'

Electrified silence. Then he banged his head. Then he looked at me again.

    IB: 'I know.'

Long silence.

    VS: 'It is hard trying to find your mum and dad when you don't know what they look like, what their names are.'

Silence.

    VS: 'You want to be a little boy in a family with a mum and dad like other children, not a man of 40 who does not know if he will ever find them.'

He burst into tears.

    IB: 'Stupid little boy crying for his mum and dad. Stupid little boy at 4 crying for his mum and dad, at 5 crying for his mum and dad, at 6 crying for his mum and dad, at 7 crying for his mum and dad.'

He began a repetitive sequence which I interrupted.

    VS: 'Isaac, every year you cried for your mum and dad and perhaps now you are going to have your own home it makes you think of them even more.'

    IB: 'Yes.'

    VS: 'And then you hate that little boy, you, who is not going to have his dream come true.'

    IB: 'I want to strangle that little boy, kill him.'

He held his hands up and mimed strangling himself.

    VS: 'So when you see the little boys at shops or out walking that aren't with a mum or dad they make you think of you.'

Long silence.

    IB: 'If I kill the little boy he won't need a mum or dad and then I can marry anyone.'

VS: 'Ah!'

I was quite amazed by this.

IB: 'You see – can't marry your mum or dad – the bible says.'

VS: 'I see – so if there is no little boy with a mum or dad then it is safe to marry anyone.'

Long silence.

IB: 'Yes. I have to marry the little boy or kill him.'

There was a painful pause.

IB: 'Muhammad says look after children. Don't kill them. His dad died and Jesus' dad killed him.'

VS: 'So you can be like Jesus' dad. So there is a bit of you that is a cruel Daddy God and a little you who is going to be killed like Jesus.'

IB: 'And then he comes alive again at Easter and I marry him.'

I thought of the way serial killers also carry a hope of being reborn in the death of their victims. However, that moment of freedom only lasts a short time.

IB: 'That murdered boy, that boy – Bulger boy. [*A little boy taken away by two older boys from a busy shopping centre in the UK and killed in 1993.*] His mum did not look after him properly. And he was a stupid boy to go off with strange boys.'

VS: 'So you are cross with the boy and his mum.'

IB: 'Yes.'

VS: 'So perhaps you are cross with the baby you for making a noise that a policeman heard and with your parents for leaving you.'

IB: 'Fuck mum and dad – stupid fuckers.'

VS: 'They were stupid fuckers because they did not think about what they were doing. They made you when they were not able to be a proper mum and dad.'

IB: 'They weren't proper.'

VS: 'They weren't. I agree.'

IB: 'And you can't marry your parents.'

VS: 'No.'

IB: 'My parents could be dead, in another country, murdered, anywhere. Could be divorced. Maybe even didn't know each other. Could be anyone. Anyone old enough. Maureen's daughter had a baby at 14, she did. Fourteen.'

VS: 'So only children under 14 are young enough to not be parents.'

IB: 'They are safe. Unless their mums don't protect them. Put them in a dustbin. [*Giggles.*] Put the lid on.'

COMMENT

Isaac did well in psychotherapy and was able to live safely in a semi-secure environment.

His impact on me was ongoing. I had never until this session considered the possibility of paedophilia and/or child murder as a defence against incest in a person who did not know their biological origin.

His use of religious references took me on another journey. Muhammad was an orphan and the very pledge of allegiance given to him by his nucleus of 12 men at Mecca included that they should not steal, commit fornication or kill their offspring. He also made quite clear that girl children were daughters of Allah and should not be cast out at birth to die. His father died a few months before he was born and therefore he was very aware of the position of orphans. Compare this with the historically and psychologically earlier position of the biblical Abraham and Isaac (Genesis 22, 1–24):

> The time came when God put Abraham to the test. 'Abraham,' he called and Abraham replied: 'Here I am.' God said: 'Take your son Isaac, your only son whom you love and go to the land of Moraih. There you shall offer him as a sacrifice on one of the hills which I will show you.' So Abraham rose early in the morning and saddled his ass. He took with him two of his men and his son Isaac and he split the firewood for the sacrifice and set out for the place of which God had spoken… There Abraham built an altar and arranged the wood. He bound his son Isaac and laid him on the altar on top of the wood. Then he stretched out his

hand and took the knife to kill his son; but the angel of the Lord called to him from heaven 'Abraham, Abraham.'

He answered: 'Here I am.' The angel of the Lord said: 'Do not raise your hand against the boy. Do not touch him. Now I know that you are a god-fearing man. You have not withheld from me your only son.' Abraham looked up and there he saw a ram caught by its thorns in a thicket. So he went and took the ram and offered it as a sacrifice instead of his son.

Abraham was willing to sacrifice his child but God allows him to desist from this and substitute an animal.

Perhaps too it was no accident that Isaac did not kill the child he had access to. He stopped just short of murder. His parents had left him for dead but had not actually murdered him. Luckily, the nature of his identification was at that moment similar.

It was only in AD 374 that infanticide began to be considered as an act of murder. Yet even then it was more out of worry for the parent's soul rather than for the child. Fear of future incest was one reason given. Saint Justin Martyr said a Christian shouldn't expose his children (the main way of causing infant death) in case they might later meet in a brothel (De Mause 1974). Abandoned children were often raised for prostitution.

Stekel (1967) saw the suicidal child as wanting to rob 'his parents of their greatest, most treasured possession: his own life.' The child knows that he will thereby inflict the greatest pain. Thus the punishment the child imposes upon himself is simultaneously the punishment he imposes on the instigator of his sufferings.

For Isaac, his parents did not value his life but he found a curious adaptation. He could identify with the absent persecuting objects in wishing to kill himself, projected into a vulnerable neglected child. As the blue-eyed dustbin baby he had a suicidal introject (Kahr 1993). By having internalised such a death wish he gives himself a momentary illusion of having found his parents. In the moment of being them he is joined with the child him in a deadly triangle. However, the same economic destructive wish also protects him from the fear of incest. A child could not be his father or mother. What are the psychobiological consequences of not knowing what your parents look like?

There is a further tragedy for the intellectually disabled individual. The societal death-wish expressed through amniocentesis and abortion when carrying a disabled baby creates a climate in which terror of being murdered further flourishes.

REFERENCES

Breen, T. and Turk, V. (1991) *Sexual Offending Behaviour by People with Learning Disabilities: Prevalence and Treatment.* Unpublished paper, University of Canterbury.

De Mause, L. (1974) *The History of Childhood.* New York: Psychohistory Press.

de Zulueta, F. (1993) *The Traumatic Roots of Destructiveness: From Pain to Violence.* London: Whurr.

Gilby, R., Wolf, L. and Goldberg, B. (1989) 'Mentally retarded adolescent sex offenders. A survey and pilot study.' *Canadian Journal of Psychiatry 34*, 542–548.

Griffiths, D., Hingsburger, D. and Christian, R. (1985) 'Treating developmentally handicapped sexual offenders: the York behaviour management services treatment program.' *Psychiatric Aspects in Mental Retardation Reviews 4*, 49–52.

Kahr, B. (1993) 'Ancient infanticide and modern schizophrenia: the clinical uses of psychohistorical research.' *Journal of Psychohistory 20*, 267–273.

Sinason, V. (1992) *Mental Handicap and the Human Condition: New Approaches from the Tavistock.* London: Free Association Books.

Sinason, V. (1996) 'From Abused to Abuser.' In C. Cordess and M. Cox (eds) *Forensic Psychotherapy: Crime, Psychodynamics and the Offender Patient.* London: Jessica Kingsley Publishers.

Sinason, V. (2004) *Learning Disability as Trauma.* Ph.D. Thesis. St George's Hospital Medical School Library.

Sinason, V. (2011) *Mental Handicap and the Human Condition.* Revised 23rd edition. London: Free Association Books.

Stekel, W. (1967) 'Symposium on Suicide.' In P. Friedman (ed.) *On Suicide.* New York: International Universities Press.

Stoller, R. (1975) *Perversion: The Erotic Form of Hatred.* London: Karnac.

Chapter 12

THE BEREAVED FAMILIES FORUM
Finding the Other Within[1]

Pam Kleinot

In this chapter Pam Kleinot takes us into the midst of a very different kind of milieu as she describes her encounter with the Bereaved Families Forum where Israeli and Palestinians come together, to share the violent loss of their loved ones through killing. There is a clear analogy to the forensic setting in that acts of the most severe violence have taken place from which both victims and perpetrators need to recover. Linking to the various accounts of such processes in the chapters of Aiyegbusi, Corbett, Adshead and Motz in particular, Kleinot explores the violence of the projection into the other across a borderline, with implicit reference to the stand-offs between the problematic pairings of both staff and patients and staff and management. She offers an account of how bereaved families are able to meet across the war zones to share their grief, no longer viewing one another as the enemy; and of how the families can see the victim within the perceived perpetrators, making it possible for the task of mourning and reparation to begin.

INTRODUCTION

> Those who cannot remember the past are doomed to repeat it.

> Santayana

Behind every act of violence, there is pain – an undigested trauma; an unmourned loss. Traumatised people unable to tell their stories through words may unconsciously communicate their narratives through enactments. The trauma is concealed in the pain and loss of buried memory. This evokes feelings of helplessness and rage. Violence is

---

1   This chapter is a revised version of the paper 'Transgenerational Trauma and Forgiveness: Looking at the Israeli-Palestinian Families Forum through a Group-Analytic Lens' that appeared in *Group Analysis 44*, 1, 97–111 (2011).

used to ward off feelings of shame. Parents unable to mourn horrific experiences may unconsciously transmit them to their children and pass the trauma from one generation to the next. This is true of individuals and societies that have suffered massive trauma.

Forgiveness and its allied concept of reconciliation is a way of metabolising aggression. This chapter is about a group of Israelis and Palestinians who have come together to work for peace after losing a family member, usually a child, in the conflict. The group is called the Bereaved Families Forum (BFF) and is made up of around 500 families. Members have had to work through their difficult feelings of hatred and revenge and find a way to work together as they are desperate to stop the cycle of violence.

I encountered the BFF while doing research in Israel. As the grandchild of persecuted Jews who fled Eastern Europe I never knew much about what had happened to them. My family never spoke about their experiences. How does one make sense of these unspoken, undigested traumas passed down from generation to generation? This is part of my own lost collective memory. I wanted to understand the escalating violence in the Middle East. I wanted to explore the appalling things that were being done to Palestinians, such as former Prime Minister Itzak Rabin ordering troops to break the bones of Palestinian children rebelling against the Occupation. Nothing prepared me for the squalor and suffering I witnessed in refugee camps in Nablus and Tul Karem. I stood at checkpoints and saw the humiliation caused to Palestinians as Israeli soldiers turned ambulances away and made people wait for hours. I struggled with feelings of disgust as well as a fear of identifying with the victim and wanting to shake off the injustices committed in my name.

I attended a meeting in Jerusalem in 2004 where an Israeli and Palestinian each told their story of losing a family member in the conflict and how they joined the BFF.

Rami Alhanan, a devoted Israeli Zionist, whose grandparents perished in the death camps during the Second World War, told of his vengeful feelings after his 14-year-old daughter was killed by a suicide bomber while shopping with friends in Jerusalem. Adel Misk, a Palestinian neurologist, described his rage after his 72-year-old father was shot by a settler and how difficult it was to face his father's killer in court. Both said they had paid the highest price imaginable in the conflict. The only way forward was to reconcile and work together for peace:

Talking allows us to move beyond our anger... If I know what's going on with you, I can understand you better and you will understand me. This is what's missing. We, the two populations, live so close to one another, we live inside one another so to speak, but we do not know each other. We need to understand that you suffer and I suffer... We have the same blood, the same pain and the same future... (Adel Misk, meeting, Jerusalem, 2004)

There is a vast amount of psychoanalytic literature on violence and revenge, but the word forgiveness is relatively absent. Although there is an absence of explicit writing, Klein (1937) and Winnicott's (1948) work on the centrality of reparation suggest that they value the capacity to forgive as an important signal of psychological health. 'The attainment of a capacity for making reparation in respect of personal guilt is one of the most important steps in the development of the healthy human being' (Winnicott 1948, p.91). The most comprehensive psychoanalytic review of the subject is by Akhtar (2002) who distinguishes between authentic and pseudo forgiveness. Premature forgiveness may be a way of avoiding hurt and anger to cope with difficult feelings.

I visited the family of a suicide bomber who had blown up a bus with 23 people in Tel Aviv. His brother, aged about 11, proudly said: 'It is no problem my brother die [sic] and go to heaven. He kills the Jews in Israel. I want all the Jews in Israel to be killed.' It was a chilling moment. I felt annihilated. The core of who I am had been assaulted... I recalled children in a refugee camp telling me that they wanted to be 'martyrs' (suicide bombers). I felt a traitor, an accomplice who shared this hatred and had betrayed my people because I had strong feelings about what was being done to Palestinians.

I was surprised when a human rights rabbi told me that 'as long as there is a Jewish State, there will be no peace... Jews are too attached to their victimhood and victims don't forgive.' This profound encounter prompted me to search my soul and understand what it meant for me: as a Jew with the Holocaust etched on my psyche, will I ever be able to forgive? As a South African, will I ever be forgiven for benefiting from apartheid because I was white and privileged?

During my research I learnt what it meant to be a witness, recognising 'Otherness'. The philosopher Margalit (2002) coined the term 'moral witness' to describe witnessing as a social function that affects collective memory. It is important to remember. Hitler used past events to shape his policies. As he invaded Poland in 1939, he ordered the mass extermination of its inhabitants, commenting, 'Who, after all, speaks today of the annihilation of the Armenians?'[2] This is inscribed on one of the walls of the US Holocaust Memorial Museum in Washington DC.

HEALING A SPLIT

When a society goes through massive trauma, it is engraved in the memory of its populations for generations and impacts on behaviour (Weinberg 2003). Israel was established as a state as a result of the Holocaust and is sensitive to threats to its security, unconsciously seeing them as threats of annihilation. I suggest that this anxiety is malignantly mirrored (Zinkin 1983) in Palestinians and the two sub-groups are in bondage with one another, trapped in an uncontrollable attractive-destructive interaction. Both feel victimised and blame each other.

An example of how the forum attempts to heal the split between Israelis and Palestinians is illustrated in a campaign to raise public awareness which was given by a bereaved father whose daughter was killed by a suicide bomber. He said:

> After an especially bloody day when many children were killed when a house in Gaza was bombed, we invited Palestinians to Jerusalem to donate their blood to the Israeli wounded. And we sneaked behind the lines to a Ramallah hospital, where we donated our blood to the Palestinian wounded. Later that day when the woman in the television studio asked us, 'How can you give your blood to the enemy?' we said to her: 'It is much less painful giving your blood to someone who needs it, than to spill it for nothing.'

This interaction goes to the heart of the conflict with blood being a linguistically powerful metaphor. Giving blood to the 'enemy' implies reparation.

I interviewed seven members of the forum, including the founder, Yitzak Frankenthal, a religious orthodox Jew whose son was kidnapped and murdered by Hamas in 1994 while serving in the Israeli army. He said: 'We don't only share the land, we share the graves of our children beneath the land.'

Frankenthal's single sentence encapsulates the essence of the conflict and the foundation of the Forum in two graphic words – land and

---

2   The mass killing of Armenians by Ottoman Turks during World War I is often referred to as the 'forgotten genocide'.

graves. The battle is over land, two sub-groups torn apart, and graves represent death, the cost of the land. Boundaries created, then children's spilt blood. Use of the word 'share' is pertinent to the bereaved families' struggle and implies sibling rivalry between the Jews and Palestinians, both descendants of Abraham. Their hatred and conflict is expressed through fighting over biblical land. Much of Genesis in the Old Testament is a discourse on sibling rivalry in which Jews and Arabs remain enemies. Their feuds may reflect the bitter hatred between their mothers thousands of years before.

The Forum was set up during South Africa's Truth and Reconciliation Commission (TRC). Although Frankenthal was influenced by it, he is adamant that the TRC was based on the Christian ethic of forgiveness which does not apply to Islam and Judaism where there is 'an eye for an eye'.

Both sides feel they are victims and after suffering years of persecution the Israelis and Palestinians cannot see themselves as abusers. However, the line between victim and perpetrator is blurred as the victim is in the perpetrator who has built a pseudo-identity of being violently tough to protect against vulnerability. The smallest humiliation is experienced as a terrible trauma-evoking panic – a fear of annihilation – which triggers violence. Hence the repetitive pattern of revenge and retaliation is established.

Frankenthal describes how the dynamics of the army in the Occupied Territories was 'anti-Jewish' and stressed that the only way to stop the hatred and bloodshed was to bring the two sides together to talk. As a matter of course, Frankenthal apologised about the Occupation to Palestinians who joined the Forum. Apology conveys remorse for something, an acknowledgment, and is linked to the ability to experience guilt and ambivalence, which Winnicott describes as the most important development in an individual related to the capacity for reparation (1958, pp.23–24). The superego is the conscience or internal moral judge (Freud 1923). There are several types of pathological superego development found in violent people including an invincible self that defends against helpless and vulnerable feelings (Parsons and Dermen 1999). In other words, a violent person with a harsh superego feels deeply persecuted and easily shamed. Tyranny is the only way of being in control, making it difficult to identify with the 'enemy' who is helpless and suffering too.

Reflecting on his own history, Frankenthal warns that many Palestinians would lose their status as Jerusalem citizens:

In Germany it was a selection to kill the Jews. Israel is making a selection to move the Palestinians out, to transfer them. We as Jewish people behave to the Palestinians exactly as we have suffered 2000 years in the Diaspora.

Use of the word 'selection' conjures up images of the death camps. In this case Israel is making a selection to transfer Palestinians out of the way. Frankenthal is tacitly talking about a repetition by making the Palestinians refugees. This may be understood as the Israelis' undigested experience of being persecuted refugees that is being projected into Palestinians who have been displaced from their homes and made refugees. Undigested experiences being re-enacted can be linked to Lloyd deMause's (1990) work on Germans' abuse of Jews as mirrors of their own traumatic childhood experience. DeMause argues that children are used as receptacles of parents' unacceptable impulses. This need for 'poisonous containers' has its roots in unfulfilled psychological needs.

The violence can be understood in terms of identification with the aggressor (Freud 1936) as well as an unconscious need to avoid feeling vulnerable. The person (or society in this context) defends itself against overwhelming helplessness and the terror of annihilation by taking on the attacking role. In other words, after centuries of persecution Israelis live under constant fear of another holocaust and perceive every threat as a risk to its survival. Like a child that has experienced early nurturing failure it lacks an adequately flexible internal protective membrane (Parsons and Dermen 1999) that would help it to register anxiety as a danger signal and make use of appropriate defences. Instead Israel has developed a rigid protective barrier, like an impenetrable fortress, and reacts violently.

I will give two vignettes from interviews I conducted that illustrate that the BFF is a microcosm of the environment in which it functions:

VIGNETTE 1: VISITING A PALESTINIAN HOME

In this example, I will show the power of the group as a transformational space when members of the Forum visited a Palestinian activist's home in Hebron after his brother was killed by a soldier at a checkpoint. Ali Abu Awwad, a convicted 'terrorist' who spent four years in an Israeli prison for his resistance activities, grew up in a politically active family and threw stones at soldiers as a teenager. He was shot by a settler during the first Intifada. His mother was a leader of Fatah, the military wing of the Palestinian Liberation Organisation. Although Ali was reluctant to meet the Forum because he believed he would be compromising his principles, he describes his experience during the meeting of around 20 people at his home with his mother and brother:

> I saw Israeli people crying in our home. I hadn't seen the tears of Israelis before… I saw the checkpoints… I saw bullets… I saw many things… I didn't see the pain or suffering of the other side… My mother started talking and she also cried. At the end, all of the people had tears in their eyes.

Ali describes the moment of being able to recognise the pain of The Other, giving him a sense of connectedness and empathic identification. Tears in the eyes of the Israeli contrast to his view of the soldier armed with guns, tanks and bullets who controls his life through checkpoints and curfews. The experience of tears in Ali's home was a moment of meeting that struck a chord between 'the enemies'.

What happened in the group is what Group Analyst Pat de Maré (Maré, Piper and Thompson 1991) called 'Koinonia', the use of dialogue to transform hate in a median group (15 to 40 people) and provides a space where new connections can be made and new meanings found. Koinonia is the anglicisation of a Greek word that means communion by intimate participation.

A process of mourning could only begin as the two sides were able to humanise each other, which is a major step in conflict resolution and marks a significant shift in dealing with pain. It is easier to express pain through violence than to feel sadness and shame. In other words, aggression can be used to mask pain, by taking revenge on those who are perceived to be responsible for the suffering.

VIGNETTE 2: CAPTURING THE ASPIRATIONAL DREAM

Israeli Zionist, Rami Alhanan, whose grandparents were killed in Auschwitz, was full of hatred and wanted revenge after his 14-year-old daughter was killed by a suicide bomber while shopping with friends in Jerusalem. He was hesitant about joining the Forum and reluctantly went to a meeting which he describes as follows:

I never saw many Arabs in my life. And I saw this amazing sight of bereaved Palestinian families coming down from the bus to make peace. I remember seeing an old Arab lady in a long black dress with a picture of a six-year-old kid on her chest. I went crazy… I cannot explain what happened…but I know this: from that moment on I have devoted my life to go from person to person, anywhere, any way, everywhere, to convey a very basic and simple truth: We are not doomed. It is not our destiny to keep on dying here forever in this holy land. We can change it. We can break this endless cycle of violence. If the two sides dig into their sins, they have both earned the right to sit on the bench of war criminals in The Hague. You won't find many cases in history where two parties on different sides of a conflict reach out for one another and talk about a better future…

Rami's account captures the aspirational – the shared and sacred – dream of two opposing sides reaching out to one another for a better future. He was moved by the woman with a picture of a child on her chest. He has taken the lost object of his daughter inside himself which has kept alive his anger and hatred. He could identify with the old woman getting off the bus – she too was carrying around a dead child. He feels connected to her. They have both lost a child. He could share her pain, shifting him from hatred and revenge. In Freud's seminal paper on 'Mourning and Melancholia' (1917) he argued that pathological mourning results from ambivalence toward the lost object. Mitscherlich and Mitscherlich's *The Inability to Mourn* (1967) marked a significant step towards the German people's confrontation with their past. They argued that unless people confronted the past and worked through what happened they could not move forward.

The Forum has to be understood in the context of a historical struggle of two traumatised-regressed people caught up in international politics. Violence is the currency and may be seen as an attempted solution to overwhelming trauma that the individual (and society) cannot process. Aggression and conflict protect against psychic pain. Defences used for this protection include splitting, dissociation and displacement.

TRANSGENERATIONAL TRAUMA

These defences are all implicated in undigested experiences and the transgenerational transmission of trauma: this links with Foulkes' (1975) concept of the foundation matrix based on the unconscious transmission of values and customs through culture across generations. There is a vast amount of literature on transgenerational trauma and silence connecting to Bruno Bettelheim's (1961) notion that 'what cannot be put into words cannot be put to rest'. Gampel (2000) has compared massive social violence to radioactivity which is impossible to stop.

The phenomenon of violence and trauma of parents being repeated in the next generation was first articulated by Selma Fraiberg. She postulated 'ghosts in the nursery' (Fraiberg, Adelson and Shapiro 1975) to describe elements of a parent's past transmitted to the infant. She referred to the unconscious presence of ghosts hovering in the nursery whereby the infant becomes the recipient of parents' feelings and expectations.

Drawing on the concept of the Social Unconscious, based on shared traumatic memories transmitted through the generations, Vamik Volkan's notion of a chosen trauma (1999, 2005) can be seen as a defence against the unbearable shame of collective humiliation. Chosen trauma refers to a major traumatic event in the nation's past that has not been mourned because it was too humiliating and it is ashamed of its defeat. The trauma lives on accompanied by an entitlement to revenge and becomes a reference point – a marker – which is deposited in future generations. The chosen trauma is reactivated when the nation faces new conflicts with enemies. The anguish of mourning is deflected through hostility and aggression.

Massive social trauma as a process that becomes encapsulated has been described by Hopper (2003). The fear of annihilation is a response to the experience of profound helplessness arising from loss following trauma.

Parents who have suffered massive social trauma and have not been able to speak about what happened may unconsciously transmit these undigested experiences to their children. The children grow up with emotionally unavailable parents and are left with a lack. This gap in experience is expressed by Boulanger (2006) about people who have 'received trauma', passed down from parents or even grandparents. The aim of psychoanalytic therapy is to make meaning of parents' emotional unavailability and to use fantasy to construct an understanding of the blank space by grafting words on to the silence. She distinguishes between two different groups: the first is growing up with a parent survivor, in which a child's personality is constructed by that parent's undigested experience of trauma and shaped by the parent's failure to reflect on their experience; the second is a person who has faced massive psychic trauma directly.

Krystal (1968) refers to massive social trauma in which an individual's personality has been shattered by the encounter with near death. He distinguishes between children and adults, pointing out that adults retreat from the sense of helplessness in terrifying situations by numbing themselves whereas children are overwhelmed by the intolerable affect. This links with Green's seminal paper on 'The Dead Mother' (1980) in which he considers the hole left after being abandoned by a mother as psychic death.

Although there is a wealth of literature concerning the Jews, there is little on the Palestinians. Gaza psychiatrist Eyad al-Sarraj (2004) says that the long history of military occupation in which children have witnessed the humiliation of their fathers has produced a 'long queue of young people willing to join the road to heaven by becoming suicide bombers'. He says:

> To understand why Palestinians are blowing themselves up in Israeli restaurants and buses is to understand the environment that produces human bombs. What propels people into such action is a long history of humiliation and a desire to revenge which every Arab harbours.

GROUP ANALYSIS

Looking at the Forum in terms of group analytic theory, communication is a key concept and is used to keep people talking, not fighting and killing each other. Foulkes viewed groups as a communicational network in which individuals were nodal points and the social permeated the individual to the core. He defined health as the free flow of communication through the network (the community). Ill health was a blockage in the system which he termed 'the autistic symptom… It mumbles to itself secretly, hoping to be overheard' (Foulkes and Anthony 1957, p.259).

The violence in the Middle East may be understood as an 'autistic symptom' and in this account it is rooted on the one side in the traumata associated with Israel's War of Independence together with the experience of near annihilation in the Holocaust; and on the other, the 1948 great disaster for Palestinians known as the Nakba. This is Arabic for 'catastrophe' and refers to the experience of Palestinians being massacred and driven out of their homes during the formation of the

State of Israel. The trauma of these experiences on both sides has not been sufficiently digested. Members of the BFF enter the group with unconscious cultural histories and shared traumatic memories of the Holocaust and Nakba. All of these issues contribute to the matrix of the Family Forum in which the Social Unconscious forms the background to each individual's pain and loss.

DISCUSSION

Racism is the emotional investment of hatred of the Other – enacting some desire without which the psyche would feel depleted (Frosh 2005). The denigrated Other carries unwanted parts of ourself – the hated and feared elements of self put into the Other. The Palestinians become the repository for what is projected into them and poisons the world around. The Palestinians also project their hatred into the Israelis and in some instances do not distinguish Jews from Israeli Jews. The Forum tries to detoxify this poison (murderous rage) by talking, witnessing and processing the pain. The unconscious Other (foreigner) is inside all of us in the form of unconscious longings (see also Chapter 2).

Both examples, that of Ali meeting Israelis in his house and that of Rami watching the Palestinians coming down from the bus, deploy the group analytic concept of mirroring whereby a person reacts to repressed parts of himself present in another and is able to re-integrate them within the self. Groups are particularly effective in processing mourning as they are based on the mirroring function (Foulkes 1964) in which the person experiencing loss needs to be acknowledged by people in a similar situation.

In the same way that wars mirror conflicts inside nations, the Forum is a mirror to the world around it. The group provides a space for a variety of mirrors to help members navigate their way through the destructive-malignant aspects of the two sides. They are able to see the pain reflected in each other's eyes and realise that both sides are suffering.

The concept of malignant mirroring (Zinkin 1983) could be deployed to understand the uncontrollable, attractive-destructive interaction between the Israelis and Palestinians who blame each other. They have to get rid of unbearable feelings of what they see in the other that they don't like in themselves. They are fascinated and repelled by each other in a highly charged context which can change with dialogue (see also Chapter 6).

The idea of hate as a source of energy that can be converted into thinking was documented by de Maré *et al.* (1991) who believed it was important to stay with the hate and keep talking in a median group. When a group starts to think together the atmosphere changes – it becomes more friendly, 'koinonia' develops and dialogue becomes possible. 'The energy of the superego is said to be derived from the Id, but we emphasize that this energy is not direct and biological, but is the frustrated energy of hate, which can become transformed into mental energy' (pp.124–125).

CONCLUSION

Group analytic thinking goes beyond the small therapeutic group and can be applied in the much wider context of the Bereaved Families Forum within the Israel-Palestine struggle as a way of understanding the process of reconciliation. Social trauma produces unresolved mourning, which can only reach resolution through the creation of a healing narrative via containment and mirroring in the group within the wider social context. The Forum is a powerful example of how bringing two conflict-ridden sides together to talk can produce a type of transformation in the group. Dialogue is an attempt to work through undigested experiences in a traumatised society. It puts in place psychological mechanisms that can provide constructive (communicational) rather than destructive acts committed in the name of war (the 'anti-group': Nitsun 1996). If internal destructiveness cannot be managed within the psyche, it leads to forms of externalisation and cycles of violence.

The Forum effectively offers a space to work through traumatic events and for two polarised groups to face The Other's suffering. Acknowledging each other's pain replaces blame. Both sides recognise that they have agency and can play a role in restoring peace. The forum offers a symbolic demonstration of the commitment to mutual recognition of acknowledging and apologising for acts of injustice and infliction of suffering. It is a practical demonstration of the process of reconciliation where action is replaced by thinking and reflection.

REFERENCES

Akhtar, S. (2002) 'Forgiveness: origins, dynamics, psychopathology, and technical relevance.' *Psychoanalytic Quarterly 71*, 2, 175–212.

Bettelheim, B. (1961) *The Informed Heart*. London: Granada.

Boulanger, G. (2006) Personal communication.

De Maré, P., Piper, R. and Thompson, S. (1991) *Koinonia: From Hate through Dialogue, to Culture in the Large Group*. London: Karnac.

DeMause, L. (1990) 'The history of child assault.' *The Journal of Psychohistory 18*, 1, 1–29.

Foulkes, S.H. (1964) *Therapeutic Group Analysis*. London: George Allen & Unwin.

Foulkes, S.H. (1975) *Group Analytic Psychotherapy, Method and Principles*. London: Gordon & Breach.

Foulkes, S.H. and Anthony, E.J. (1957) *Group Psychotherapy: the Psychoanalytic Approach*. Harmondsworth: Penguin.

Foulkes, S.H. and Anthony, E.J. (1965) *Group Psychotherapy: the Psychoanalytic Approach*. (Second Edition). Harmondsworth: Penguin. London: Karnac.

Fraiberg, S., Adelson, E. and Shapiro, V. (1975) 'Ghosts in the nursery: A psychoanalytic approach to the problems of impaired infant-mother relationships.' *Journal of the American Academy of Child Psychiatry 14*, 387–422.

Freud, A. (1936) *The Ego and the Mechanisms of Defence*. London: Hogarth.

Freud, S. (1917) 'Mourning and Melancholia.' In R. Frankel (ed.) *Essential Papers on Object Loss*. New York: New York University Press.

Freud, S. (1923) *The Ego and the Id*. New York: W.W. Norton.

Frosh, S. (2005) *Hate and the 'Jewish Science': Anti-Semitism, Nazism and Psychoanalysis*. Houndmills, Basingstoke, Hampshire and New York: Palgrave Macmillan.

Gampel, Y. (2000) 'The Prevalence of the Uncanny in Social Violence.' In A.C.G.M. Robben and M.M. Suárez-Orozco (eds) *Cultures under Siege: Collective Violence and Trauma* (Publication of the Society for psychological Anthropology). Cambridge: Cambridge University Press.

Green, A. (1980) 'The Dead Mother.' Reprinted in A. Green (1986) *On Private Madness*. London: Hogarth Press.

Hopper, E. (2003) 'Incohesion: Aggregation/Massification; the Fourth Basic Assumption in the Unconscious Life of Groups and Group-like Social Systems.' In R. Lipgar and M. Pines (eds) *Building on Bion: Roots*. London: Jessica Kingsley Publishers.

Klein, M. (1937) 'Love, Guilt and Reparation.' In *Melanie Klein: Love, Guilt and Reparation and Other Works 1921–1945*. London: Hogarth.

Krystal, H. (ed.) (1968) *Massive Psychic Trauma*. New York: International Universities Press.

Margalit, A. (2002) *The Ethics of Memory*. Cambridge, MA: Harvard University Press.

Mitscherlich, A. and Mitscherlich, M. (1975) *The Inability to Mourn*. New York: Grove Press.

Nitsun, M. (1996) *The Anti-group: Destructive Forces in the Group and their Creative Potential*. London: Routledge.

Parsons, M. and Dermen, S. (1999) 'The Violent Child and Adolescent.' In M. Lanyado and A. Horne (eds) *The Handbook of Child and Adolescent Psychotherapy: Psychoanalytic Perspectives*. London: Routledge.

Sarraj, E. (2004) Faculty for Israeli-Palestinian Peace Conference, Jerusalem. Unpublished lecture.

Volkan, V. (1999). 'Psychoanalysis and diplomacy: Part I. Individual and large group identity.' *Journal of Applied Psychoanalytic Studies 1*, 29–55.

Volkan, V. (2005). 'Large-group identity, large-group regression and massive violence. Group-analytic contexts.' *International Newsletter of Group Analytic Society 30*, 8–26.

Weinberg, H. (2003). 'The Culture of the Group and Groups from Different Cultures.' *Group Analysis 36*, 2, 253–268.

Winnicott, D.W. (1948) 'Reparation in Respect of Mother's Organized Defence against Depression.' In *Through Paediatrics to Psycho-Analysis: Collected Papers* (1992). London: Karnac.

Winnicott, D.W. (1958) 'Psycho-Anlysis and the Sense of Guilt.' In *The Maturational Process and the Facilitating Environment* (1990). London: Karnac.

Zinkin, L. (1983) 'Malignant mirroring.' *Group Analysis 26*, 2, 113–126.

Chapter 13

WHAT MAKES A SECURE SETTING SECURE?[1]

Stanley Ruszczynski

In this chapter Stanley Ruszczynski presents the many challenges that face institutions designed to deal with forensic patients. His is the first of three closing chapters in this volume, each concerned with the ways in which individual practitioners and staff teams can have some of their own specific needs thought about and addressed. Ruszczynski writes of the need to preserve psychoanalytic understanding while retaining a setting that is secure and responsive to the particular needs and social circumstances of this group, working in organisations and institutions where there is much need for resilience, little space for reflection and continual demand to show courage under fire.

INTRODUCTION

In this chapter I offer an understanding of the culture of secure settings, how this inevitably impacts on all levels of staff who work in these institutions, and discuss suggestions about the therapeutic value of paying close attention to the emotional states and behaviours that get generated in these environments. I discuss the importance of providing regular and consistent multi-disciplinary staff groups to provide opportunities for colleagues to reflect on their experiences of working with their patients so that some of the disturbances in the patient's mind and behaviour will be processed, understood and be better attended to. These reflective practice groups will also help process the inevitable disturbances generated in the staff, who are then less likely to get caught up in possible unconscious enactments

---

1   This chapter is a revised version of a discussion paper, titled 'Boundaries and Culture', originally presented to the Clinical Security Practice Forum at the Department of Health in February 2011. Parts of it have been previously published in Ruszczynski (2008).

through poor care provision, malpractice, boundary violations and other professional failures.

This discussion is based on my experience of consulting to multi-disciplinary teams, single discipline groups and managers in high, medium and low secure settings, in prisons and in community services. This consultative work is grounded in long-term, in-depth clinical work with forensic and personality disordered patients, undertaken at the Portman Clinic (Tavistock and Portman NHS Foundation Trust), London, an NHS outpatient psychotherapy clinic.

High secure settings are responsible for the management, care and, when possible, treatment of extremely difficult and often very disturbing patients and offenders. These patients/offenders are largely defined by their antisocial behaviour that is damaging (physically and psychologically) to the victim(s) and often the perpetrators themselves. These may be acts of delinquency, criminality, physical and sexual violence or sexual perversion – and often a combination of such acts. In addition to their disordered personality, sometimes diagnosed as antisocial personality disorder, several of these patients/offenders have a psychiatric illness. Hale and Dhar have argued that personality disorder may not infrequently be a defence against a psychotic illness (Hale and Dhar 2008).

THE IMPACT ON OTHERS

Such difficult and disturbing behaviour intrudes on other people, who, if they are the victims, are directly hurt and violated by the act(s), both physically and psychologically. Other people too, including professional staff, often feel violated by such acts, not necessarily physically but psychologically, through the emotional impact such behaviour can arouse. Staff working with these patients/offenders can often feel disturbed by what they learn of the offenders' behaviour, and by the offenders' behaviour itself which sometimes becomes enacted in the care setting. This difficulty is exacerbated when staff are working on a ward or a prison landing with a dozen or more patients/offenders, all of whom have committed acts of gross violence or sexual perversion.

One could say that 'evidence' of this difficulty is demonstrated in the fact that it is not unusual for staff to 'forget' details of the violence and perversity that resulted in their patients now being in their care. How does one keep in mind the often very disturbing, violent and perverse behaviours of the dozen or more patients/offenders one is working with every day? Surviving the working day might require staff to distance themselves from such disturbing information, but this of course has the danger of compromising both the therapeutic task and security requirements.

These ideas of intrusion and violation, and the question of how staff might be assisted to make it more possible to keep the patient and his history in mind, as well as process the information, is central to my discussion.

DISORDERED PERSONALITIES

Mentally ill patients can be seen, mostly, to have a problem with their mind – they are *mentally* ill, and we can to some degree distance ourselves from that state of mind by, for example, responding to these patients in a 'medicalised' or even 'scientific' way (Hinshelwood 1999). They have an illness, they can be diagnosed, they can be offered medication, their more obvious psychotic symptoms reduce or disappear and they are seen as having got better. Even when they have displayed disturbing, violent or perverse behaviour, that behaviour can be 'explained' as if it were due to the psychiatric illness.

By contrast, people who *act out* their difficulties in antisocial ways often have a disturbing emotional impact on those around them, making it much more difficult to distance oneself. The sense of disturbance, intrusion or violation, resulting from delinquency, criminality, violence or sexual perversions, has an inevitable impact. Strong feelings are aroused which may include disturbing feelings of condemnation, anger, fear, disgust, outrage and revenge, and the feelings are often particularly disturbing in relation to sexually violent and perverse behaviour. These toxic emotions confound and disturb thinking and possible responses. In other words, these patients/ offenders may be said to have a disturbance of social relating which has a toxic impact on those around them.

These patients/offenders are difficult because they arouse difficult feelings and hence affect attitudes towards them, and not just in society in general but also among service providers (Hinshelwood 1999; Ruszczynski 2007). Staff are professionally engaged with patients/ offenders who have brutally assaulted or murdered, or viciously sexually assaulted others. Often these patients/offenders have had similarly disturbing neglectful, abusive, violent and perverse aspects to their own early life.

Professional competence can feel undermined and even destroyed in the face of these actions. This may manifest in a failure in the capacity to think about the perpetrator with the result that the disturbing act is reacted to by punishment, incarceration or, if the patient is already in institutional care, by seclusion or by medication. Staff might act in a harsh way, even callously, as if in unthinking retaliation to the sense of being undermined or threatened. Sometimes there is an active demonisation of the perpetrator. All of these can become reinforced by the institutional practices and norms of the culture of secure settings. In addition, there may sometimes emerge feelings of excitement, curiosity and seduction.

POSSIBLE ORIGINS OF DISTURBING BEHAVIOURS

Such descriptions of these patients and offenders and the disturbances that they cause are not a criticism but an attempt to understand the meaning of their antisocial behaviour and the feelings evoked in those around them, including professionals.

Evidence of difficulties can often be traced back to early childhood. Genetics, temperament and a likely history of deprivation, rejection and cruelty all play a part. Protective factors such as caring family relationships and stable backgrounds are absent from their formative lives.

If the original family environment was one in which parental figures expressed high levels of depressive or narcissistic anxiety, aggression and/ or sexual or physical abuse towards the child, the child would not only have been deprived of parents' reflective mind as a model for developing his own, but may also have learned to actively avoid thinking about his own and others' experiences because they were disturbing or violent. As a consequence there is little likelihood of the development of either a coherent sense of self or much sense of a real other person. As a result, no system of personal or interpersonal values is likely to develop, nor a moral code by which behaviour and actions could be judged. Callousness will emerge as a way of functioning, an apparently total lack of sensitivity which is rooted in anxiety. Safety or relief is provided by a sense of triumph or dominance over the external world, or the immediate attention or admiration of others.

Further, this absence of a sufficiently attentive parental environment during early development, together perhaps with some constitutional vulnerability, results in a poorly developed capacity for reflection and emotional self-regulation. This lack of an internal capacity to manage and process anxieties, impulses and conflicts, leaves such people with no choice but to use the external space they live in, their own bodies or the bodies of other people and environment around them, as the canvas upon which they express their emotional states (Fonagy *et al.* 2002). The impact of an act of violence or sexual abuse generates toxic feelings not only in the victims but in all who come to know of these acts.

What might be more difficult to think about is that this evocation of disturbing feelings in the victim is actually the unconscious purpose of the perpetrator who needs to rid himself of correspondingly difficult feelings within himself because these feelings are felt to be unbearable and cannot be tolerated (Ruszczynski 2007). Similar processes inevitably take place, but usually in a less open and dramatic way, in relation to staff who will also be affected by offenders who unconsciously need to generate disturbed feelings in others as a way of distancing themselves from the feelings within themselves. Staff members are sometimes overtaken by these feelings causing them to behave in unacceptable ways that may lead to boundary violations.

There is clinical evidence that, for example, acts of violence are often perpetrated by offenders who feel humiliated, frightened and vulnerable. Through projective processes, these offenders are unconsciously attempting to diminish this in themselves by 'creating' in their victim, through their aggression to that victim, someone who is frightened and fearful. The paedophile, in a similar way, is creating in their victim a child who is treated in a grossly age-inappropriate way, whose generational boundaries between child and adult experiences are breached, who is invited into a deep confusion between sensual and sexual experiences, and for whom the notion of the caretaker adult is shattered. It is not unusual to often find these highly damaging experiences in the developmental history of many offenders.

There is something both inevitable and unconsciously purposeful about the disturbing and difficult behaviours enacted by patients and offenders in secure settings. These people simply are like this, it is the way they often function in all their social relationships. There are usually multiple examples of worrisome, disturbing and violating behaviours in their early history. How better to communicate an unbearable state of mind than, through unconscious projective processes, to arouse a similar state of mind in another person. This can be done by affecting the atmosphere of a relationship or by violently or perversely acting on the other person's body as well as their mind. This makes thinking difficult, which has been part of the purpose of locating these experiences outside of the mind.

THE CULTURE OF SECURE SETTINGS

As this way of functioning is characterological, it does not fundamentally change when these patients or offenders come into the care of the mental health or social care services or the criminal justice system. The settings which offer care, treatment, management or constraint become the arenas for this enactment. The fundamental dynamics continue to find expression in secure settings despite some limitations due to physical and procedural management.

It is likely that staff working with violent patients may feel frightened or violated (and sometimes react sadistically); those working with sexually perverse patients may feel disgusted and/or corrupted (and sometimes feel voyeuristic and seduced); those working with personality disordered patients might feel abused, hostile or omnipotently indulgent. Staff groups working with patients and offenders in secure settings are confronted with a range of patients who are likely to be all of the above: violent, sexually perverse and personality disordered. As a result, the institution is likely to be regularly affected by and the staff potentially disrupted and disturbed by fear, violation, corruption, seduction and abuse. Staff may come to feel defensively sadistic or dismissively disgusted and abusive by, for example, being inappropriately indulgent towards the patient, or simply shut off and not be able to think about the offender or his management and care (Ruszczynski 2008).

The Fallon Enquiry Report into Ashworth Hospital states: 'Dr O… gave evidence…on behalf of the Royal Collage of Psychiatrists… He invited us to pay regards to what he regarded as the "toxic emotional processes" in Special Hospitals: "We are dealing with the most disturbed individuals in society, incarcerated with each other for a very long period of time, working with staff groups who are also there for a very long period of time and there is a corrosive effect on the staff group unless in fact management is aware of this, unless all the staff groups are in touch with this"…' (Ashworth Special Hospital 1999, p.324).

Without this awareness, produced by regular opportunities to reflect on these inevitable and difficult experiences, staff working with such patients are destined to sometimes repeat their patients' early corrupt, mindless and depriving experiences. In other words, individual staff, staff groups, institutional structures and the institutions themselves all become susceptible to the enactments that are fundamental to how these patients and offenders function in their lives.

EXTENDING THE WAYS OF THINKING ABOUT MANAGEMENT AND TREATMENT OF OFFENDERS

If this is the predominant culture in secure settings, the treatment model for these patients/offenders has to be extended beyond their individual or group programmes, their occupational therapy, educational programmes and other more active interventions. It is essential that there is reflective attention on the part of the staff to the way in which the institution and those who staff it are affected by their everyday working relationship with such patients. To paraphrase Richard Lucas, who writes powerfully about 'the psychotic wavelength' (Lucas 2009), how can clinicians working with patients in secure settings 'tune into the perverse or anti-social wavelength', where disavowal and aggressive projection of unbearable feeling states into the other's mind *and body* are central dynamics both within the patient and, inevitably, within the settings and staff groups working with these patients? With the body being employed in a violent or perverse act to manage these states, by projecting them in such a concrete way into the other, the capacity to think and reflect is made especially difficult.

Managers and senior clinicians have a crucial role to play. As they have a different function in secure institutions, they may have less regular contact with offenders and therefore be less affected by these disturbing dynamics. However, if they understand that these disturbances are inevitable and have to be addressed by frontline staff as part of the management and treatment of these patients/offenders, they could ensure that opportunities for reflective examination and exploration of the culture and dynamics of the institution take place on a regular basis as a fundamental part of the treatment model.

Crucial to the development of such treatment setting and therapeutic models has to be the understanding that personality disordered patients and offenders are likely to have a disordered reaction to care due to their early life experiences. This is characterised by regular attacks, both actively and passively, on the care being provided. The attack may be by aggressively dismissive means or, more often, by corrupting the help. This is likely to be based on their personal experience of parents and other early caretakers being abusive, violent, sexually perverse, or absent and neglectful. This results in one of the most difficult aspects of what is required by the practitioner in a forensic setting. The sense of good work and of the patient 'getting better', probably desired by all clinicians, is often absent for long periods. If this 'absence' is not understood as being part of the patient's symptoms, then it can be very demoralising to the staff or can lead to the conclusion that the patient is 'not making use of treatment' (Hinshelwood 2002; Ruszczynski 2010).

For the patient who has little, if any, trust in others, aggression becomes a likely defensive posture. Equally, because of the likely history of absence of good care, a sense or even provocation of neglect also emerges. This is important to understand when, by definition, a secure institution attempts to provide both care and custody. Both care and control can become corrupted – care might become complacent or withheld and control becomes cruel and sadistic. The tension inherent in maintaining a perspective whereby both care and control are kept in mind is in danger of being lost, with the result of providing just one or the other (see Chapter 6).

Sometimes neither care nor control is provided, and the patient gets, in effect, 'forgotten' about, sometimes for a long time. This 'forgetting' in itself becomes abusive of the patient and their need, and it is likely to be a repetition of the patient's earlier experiences of being forgotten about by parents or other carers who should have kept that person in their mind but did not do so, for whatever reason. This identification with neglect, on the part of the patient, is as disruptive of establishing reasonable care as in the identification with and enactment of aggression (Ruszczynski 2010).

THE CULTURE OF ENQUIRY

If treatment services are to be further developed for these patients, as opposed to providing just containment or at worst warehousing them, it is helpful to understand that the care institution itself, the staff relationships to the patients and to each other, organisational structures and behaviours, are all likely to be affected and even corrupted by the emotionally disturbing impact generated by these patients. It is as if the institution itself comes to be in need of self-observation, containment, analysis and interpretation – that is, it needs the space and opportunity to reflect on itself and its relationships to the primary therapeutic and security task. It is in this way that the institution itself can think of itself as the 'patient' needing this attention and reflective care (Ruszczynski 2008).

If staff can sustain a thinking capacity then in doing so they provide a psychological setting within which *some* patients might be able to make the first tentative steps away from acting out their internal worlds. They may begin to be able to reflect on themselves and on their relating to others, thus developing a less disturbed and disturbing way of functioning.

The provision of an opportunity for the whole multi-disciplinary staff team to attend reflective practice groups has been found to be helpful. These groups are centred in the treatment setting, whether that be a hospital ward, prison landing, community mental health service or hostel. The task of these meetings is to share the experience of working with a particular patient. This is done by the meeting being reminded of the patient's developmental history, of the index offence or primary difficulties or symptoms, and some information about the patient's experiences with health and social care. It is stressed that the purpose of the meeting is then to discuss the patient, with each member of the team voicing his or her thoughts, feelings and experiences as openly as possible. The discussion does not have decision-making or action planning as its primary focus.

Different members of staff in these reflective practice groups are likely to be identified with and come to represent different aspects of the patient's often fragmented internal world. As these thoughts, feelings and observations about the patient are shared among the staff group in the course of the reflective practice meeting, a more comprehensive picture of the patient develops and, as a result, a more coherent picture of the patient begins to emerge. It is as if the group takes on the role of the interested 'parental mind', and begins to see the patient in a more integrated way, an experience that the patient has most probably never had. As this happens in the treatment setting, the ways in which the staff relate to the patient will now be informed by this more integrated picture of the patient who as a result, over time, may slowly begin to identify with this image of himself. Having an external consultant who is not 'caught up' with the patient in the same way as the care team are likely to be will generally facilitate this reflective process (see Chapter 14).

This activity, though it is always focused on each occasion on a particular patient, goes beyond support for working with any one patient: it also facilitates the development of a 'culture of enquiry' in the ward or on the prison landing, influencing work with all patients/ offenders in the ward or prison (Main 1983; Day and Pringle 2001).

Furthermore, this process will have an impact on the security within the setting in which the patient is being taken care of. Deeper knowledge of the patient enhances relational security if relational security is understood as an ongoing process on the part of the staff who develop a capacity to keep in their minds the patient with all his/ her complexity. This is the real value of relational security, a process whereby a patient is that bit more secure because he is related to in this more meaningful way by the staff who manage him. By stressing that a *process* is being described, recognition is given to the need for staff to be constantly monitoring their experiences with their patients and the dynamics which get generated.

Developing a skilled workforce is essential in meeting the challenges set by these patients and offenders and building upon earlier work (Department of Health 2003a, b). In 2009 the Department of Health and the Ministry of Justice jointly launched the 'Personality Disorder: Knowledge and Understanding Framework', which consists of different levels of trainings including an 'awareness level' and two more formal degree level teaching programmes that are intended significantly to enhance the competencies of those working with people suffering from personality disorder.

I have stressed in this chapter the need for staff in secure settings to 'learn about the patient' through the process of discussing and thinking about the way patients conduct themselves, how they interact with other patients and how they relate with staff. Central to this learning will be the processing of the emotional experiences generated in the staff by the patient through their behaviour and the nature of their interactions.

CONCLUSION: REFLECTIVE PRACTICE, RELATIONAL SECURITY AND ENHANCED CARE IN SECURE SETTINGS

Those working in secure institutions usually carry out difficult work with great tolerance and skill. This chapter addresses how this might be further enhanced. The assessment of, and appropriate attention to, risk and dangerousness needs to be constantly monitored in relation to these patients. In doing so, attention needs to be paid to the balance between care and control. There is a constant need to sustain physical and procedural security as well as growing recognition that the third arm of the security triangle, relational or dynamic security, needs more attention than it perhaps has received to date.

This is likely to be achieved through the development of regular and consistent opportunities for whole staff groups, together with an external consultant, to reflect together on their experiences of working with their patients, in meetings dedicated to discussing and thinking about a particular patient. By doing this, some of the disturbances in the patient's mind and behaviour will be processed, understood and will be better attended to. Equally, some of the inevitable disturbances generated in staff of secure institutions will be processed and understood and will therefore be less likely to be acted out through malpractice, boundary violations and other professional failures. These are often the products of undigested and unprocessed disturbances of the delinquent, perverse and violent dynamics inevitably present in secure settings.

REFERENCES

Ashworth Special Hospital (1999) *Report of the Committee of Inquiry, Vol.1*, January 1999.

Day, L. and Pringle, P. (2001) *Reflective Enquiry into Therapeutic Institutions*. London: Karnac.

Department of Health (2003a) *Personality Disorder: No Longer a Diagnosis of Exclusion. Policy Implementation Guidance for the Development of Services for People with Personality Disorder*. London: Department of Health.

Department of Health (2003b) *Breaking the Cycle of Rejection: The Personality Disorder Capabilities Framework*. London: Department of Health.

Fonagy, P., Gergely, G., Jurist, E. and Target, M. (2002) *Affect Regulation, Mentalisation and the Development of the Self*. New York: Other Press.

Hale, R. and Dhar, R. (2008) 'Flying a Kite – Observations on Dual (and Triple) Diagnosis.' *Criminal Behaviour and Mental Health 18*, 145–152.

Hinshelwood, R. (1999) 'The difficult patient: the role of 'scientific psychiatry' in understanding patients with chronic schizophrenia or personality disorder.' *British Journal of Psychiatry 174*, 187–190.

Hinshelwood, R. (2002) 'Abusive help – helping abuse: the psychodynamic impact of severe personality disorder on caring institutions.' *Criminal Behaviour and Mental Health 12*, S20–S30.

Lucas, R. (2009) *The Psychotic Wavelength: A Psychoanalytic Perspective for Psychiatry*. London: Routledge.

Main, T.M. (1983) 'The Concept of a Therapeutic Community: Variations and Vicissitudes.' In T. Main (ed.) (2001) *The Ailment and other Psychoanalytic Essays.* London: Karnac.

Ruszczynski, S. (2007) 'The Problem of Certain Psychic Realities: Aggression and Violence as Perverse Solutions.' In D. Morgan and S. Ruszczynski (eds) *Lectures in Violence, Perversion and Delinquency.* London: Karnac.

Ruszczynski, S. (2008) 'Thoughts from Consulting in Secure Settings: do Forensic Institutions need Psychotherapy.' In J. Gordon and G. Kirtchuk (eds) *Psychic Assaults and Frightened Clinicians: Countertransference in Forensic Settings.* London: Karnac.

Ruszczynski, S. (2010) 'Becoming Neglected: a Perverse Relationship to Care.' *British Journal of Psychotherapy 26*, 1, 22–32.

Chapter 14

THE TRAUMATISED-ORGANISATION-IN-THE-MIND
Opening Up Space for Difficult Conversations
in Difficult Places

Christopher Scanlon

In this chapter Christopher Scanlon draws upon educational, psychosocial, group analytic and systems psychodynamic theories to explore the conceptual frameworks underpinning 'team development' interventions in the organisational context. He joins with other authors in this volume to argue that the reflective capacity of the organisation is one of the markers of health and a source of resilience in the face of attack. Scanlon explores the role of the Team Development Consultant (TDC) in promoting reflective practice and suggests that s/he may need to show a particular kind of 'courage under fire' as s/he invites teams to face up to the challenges of working together in the highly stressful and contested conditions that constitute the forensic environment.

INTRODUCTION AND BACKGROUND

Ah Love, let us be true
To one another! For the world, which seems
To lie before us like a land of dreams…
Hath really neither joy, nor love, nor light,
Nor certitude, nor peace, nor help for pain:
And we are here as on a darkling plain
Swept with confused alarms of struggle and flight,
Where ignorant armies clash by night.

Excerpts from *Dover Beach*, Matthew Arnold (2004)

In considering the problematic and difficult work undertaken on our behalf by the forensic mental health system, a number of theorists have posed questions about the interpersonal and systems-psychodynamic problems at the heart of the work in terms of the 'Forensic dilemma'. I want to revisit this concept briefly at the beginning of this chapter. Bonnie Honig (1996 cited in Hoggett 2005, p.183) describes 'dilemmatic spaces' as opening up when conversations about things that do not fit together, or that contain inherent contradictions and antinomies, must take place and when actions are demanded that will inevitably disappoint someone. This is the day-to-day experience of living and working in the Forensic Mental Health system. There is a growing literature about the potentially traumatising impact of these disappointing dynamics and how they are (dis)played out at an organisational level (Aiyegbusi and Clarke 2008; Aiyegbusi and Kelly 2012; Armstrong 2005; Campling, Davies and Farquharson 2004; Cooper and Lousada 2005; Dartington 2010; Gordon and Kirtchuk 2008; Hopper 2003, 2011; Menzies-Lyth 1992; Obholzer and Roberts 1994; Scanlon and Adlam 2011a, b *inter alia*). Much of this work is based on explorations of interrelated and interacting theories of practice rooted in systems-psychodynamic, group and organisational dynamic (mis)understandings of the nature of social, structural and institutional defences against anxiety and the complex reciprocal processes that *enforce* and *reinforce* them. It is beyond the scope of this short chapter to represent this theorising in detail; except perhaps to state my own view, that 'the work' in forensic settings is *always* characterised by encounters with distress and traumatic experience that inevitably become internalised and personified by individual team members in what I am calling, with acknowledgement and respect to my colleagues David Armstrong (2005) and Earl Hopper (2003, 2011), the 'traumatised-organisation-in-the-mind'.

Bion (1975) suggested that, in order to be able to think in and about these 'dilemmatic' spaces, first we have to find ways to tolerate the experience of 'not knowing' and then to contain the emergent anxiety until such a time when something more 'thinkable' may (or may not) begin to emerge. Describing the state of mind necessary to manage this 'not knowing' Bion (1970, p.125) makes use of the term 'negative capability' – a term coined by the poet John Keats to describe a longed-for state of mind '...when a man [sic] is capable of being in uncertainties, mysteries, doubts, without any irritable reaching after reason.'

For the purposes of this chapter, I propose that to think within, and about, the potentially or actually traumatised-organisation-in-the-mind is a shared task, the responsibility for which lies not, primarily, with individuals but with the team. This is the case because the work is essentially and necessarily an *inter*-activity that is always inter-personal, inter-professional and inter-agency. To make the team the focus of attention is also to pay due respect to pervasive, (dis)organising social defences and potentially traumatising group dynamics that are at the heart of all work with difficult people in difficult places; and to acknowledge that, if we are to stand any chance of managing ourselves effectively in these difficult conversations in and about these dilemmatic spaces, we have to work together.

THE THERAPEUTIC MILIEU AND THE PSYCHOLOGICALLY INFORMED (PLANNED) ENVIRONMENT (PI(P)E)

Tom Main was one of the early pioneers of work exploring the nature of the types of therapeutic milieu that have recently been rediscovered (as if lost) under the broader rubrics of PIPEs (Psychologically Informed Planned Environments) and PIEs (Psychologically Informed Environments) (Department for Communities and Local Government 2010; Johnson and Haigh 2010). Main described a primary task of the therapeutic milieu (comprising staff and patients) as the maintenance of 'a culture of enquiry into personal, interpersonal and inter-system problems…of impulses, defences and relations as these are expressed and arranged socially' (Main 1983). In this late-modern (re)discovery of the concept it would appear that 'Psychologically Informed' is the preferred description. However, for myself I consider the emphasis on the psychological to be misleading and unhelpful. If we must have a new description for 'therapeutic milieu' (which I myself do not think necessary) I suggest that it is more helpful to use a more generic descriptive term such as 'enabling environment' (Campling *et al.* 2004; Johnson and Haigh 2011; Royal College of Psychiatrists 2010) or a description that places the emphasis upon the *collective*, the social or the group: and here I offer, somewhat ironically perhaps, 'Psychosocially Informed Environment' as a term that might (re)locate the responsibility for what takes place in the therapeutic environment firmly *between* people, rather than within their or (an)other's psychology. It also challenges any assumption that the knowledge necessary to progress this task is necessarily to be found within narrow definitions of what might constitute a 'psychological therapist'. Better still we might think about the task in terms of enabling the nurturing of a mindful or intelligent kindness (Coltart 1993; Mace 2007; Ballat and Campling 2011; see also the Foreword to this volume).

Confusingly, over the years a wide range of similar and different team-focused interventions that aim to promote this 'culture of enquiry' in staff working in therapeutic milieux have been proposed. There have been generic terms used such as Sensitivity Groups (e.g. Bramley 1990; Haigh 2000); Staff Support Groups (e.g. Kanas 1986; Novakovic 2002; Hartley and Kennard 2009; Simpson 2010); Team Development/ Consultation Groups (e.g. Carlyle and Evans 2005; Thorndycraft and McCabe 2008; Blumenthal *et al.* 2011) and more specifically 'badged' interventions such as Interpersonal Dynamics and Multidisciplinary Team Work (Reiss and Kirtchuk 2009); Interface of Meaning and Projection Formulation (IMPF) (Canning and Babb 2010) and AMBIT Mentalization Groups (Bevington and Fuggle 2012), to name but a few. Some terms, like Staff Sensitivity Groups, would seem to be out of favour whilst others, for instance Staff Support Groups, though a rather empty description of a heterogeneous range of somewhat anodyne interventions, persevere – perhaps reflecting a desire that some staff teams might prefer to be soothed and supported to carry on doing what they are already doing, rather than to be sensitised, reflected or to develop? Regardless of how these interventions are styled, although team-focused interventions are widely (though not universally) practised, the diversity and overlapping nature of many of these approaches contributes to a conceptual 'Tower of Babel' of confusions such that the epistemological frameworks underpinning them remain poorly understood. There is therefore little strategic agreement about which intervention, if any, might be better applied in which settings and by whom.

One reason for this lack of understanding is an often unspoken assumption that models of practice derived from particular psychological therapies[1] can be applied, by default, to a primary task of enhancing the therapeutic milieu within a wider culture of enquiry. This assumption, where present, is problematic in a number of ways. For example, if

---

1   I am using the term 'psychological therapies', rather than psychotherapies, so as to include a critique of interventions derived from Clinical, Counselling, Forensic, Humanistic, Integrative and Organisational Psychologies as well as a wide range of psychodynamically informed approaches – even though I would argue that some of these approaches, for example group-analysis, group-relations, systems-psychodynamic and systems-centred models, are in my view quintessentially (and helpfully) 'psychosocial' rather than 'psychological' in their approach.

the knowledge and skills necessary to progress the task are taken to be merely an extension of these different psychological therapies, does this mean that being a 'good enough' therapist is sufficient qualification? On the other hand, if the required knowledge and skills are seen as having different characteristics, what are they and how is the Team Development Consultant (TDC) to acquire, maintain and develop a working knowledge of them? It also begs a question about whether the knowledge base derived from working in general mental health settings is directly transferrable or whether, as argued by Adshead (1991), Cordess, Welldon and Riley (1994), Cordess and Cox (1996), McGauley (2002), Norton and McGauley (2000) amongst others, there is a specialised knowledge base required for understanding the interpersonal, team-based, organisational and systemic problems that are more specific to forensic settings.

My own view is that the Team Development Consultancy that I am setting out to describe here is a type of organisational research that is primarily an *educational* activity which, though it also requires extensive knowledge of a range of 'psychological approaches', is not an extension of 'psychological' work (Ruszczynski 2008). Some psychological therapists are good at it – and some, though they may be expert in their field, most definitely are not. The TDC must also have significant expert knowledge of the management issues at the heart of the forensic dilemma because it is vitally important that such work must always be in support of the wider management imperative of balancing the safety of patients (and staff) with the safety of the general public. This is not to say that the TDC must blindly support (mis)understandings of this 'management function' by any given manager, but rather that s/he must have the confidence, the seniority and the open channels of communication to be able to inform, support or challenge local decisions as the ethics of the situation demands.

To be effective, therefore, the team development group should be integrated into the life of the team and the TDC should be experienced (impossibly) as both a part of, and apart from, the team. If the TDC is experienced as apart from and positioned as an observing 'outsider' it can be very difficult to be credibly alongside and to participate actively in these difficult conversations. On the other hand, in order to be able to take up their authority and manage themselves effectively in role the TDC needs also to be sufficiently able to observe the unfolding team dynamic without being 'sucked in'. Here we might also remind ourselves that Freud (1937) suggested that there were three impossible professions: clinical practice, education and governance. In so far as this type of intervention derives its knowledge base significantly from all three of these areas, those of us who attempt to undertake these roles must have our own reflective spaces to think together about this aspect of our work, as well as about the troubled parts of our own minds that have led us to such a 'self appointed impossible task' (Roberts 1994).

Against this background, the aim of this chapter is to undertake a critical review of some relevant literature from these different practice-based disciplines. In order to be able to do this effectively I am concerned that the review be presented in an inter-professional language that might be more accessible by all – the language of *reflective practice* (Pietroni 1992). The discussion will be framed by a critical review of relevant educational literature discussing reflective practice (Schön 1983, 1987) and its contribution to the development of a more effective 'culture of enquiry'. The foreground of the discussion will be a more focused discussion of some systems-psychodynamic and group-dynamic considerations about the use of such team-focused reflective practice interventions in forensic settings.

REFLECTIVE PRACTICE AND THE NATURE OF PROFESSIONAL KNOWLEDGE

To travel hopefully is a better thing than to arrive,
and the true success is to labour.

Virginibus Puerisque, Robert Louis Stevenson (1881)

In discussing the nature of skilful practice, the educational philosopher Gilbert Ryle (1949) made the distinction between two domains of knowledge that he described as 'knowing that' and 'knowing how'. He described 'knowing that' as having more to do with 'theoretical understanding', whereas *know-how* involved what we might call the capacity to think one's own thoughts (Gabbard and Wilkinson 1994) and act accordingly whilst under fire. Schön (1983, 1987) coined the term 'knowing-in-action' to refer to such 'know-how' and he suggested that the predominant organisational and managerial paradigm, which he called the 'technical-rational' approach, takes little account of these ways of knowing. In this approach there is no thought to build in places and spaces for facilitating the acquisition and development of this 'know-how'. Rather the technical-rational perspective considers practice to be merely the application of a pre-determined body of technical knowledge that is embodied in sets of rational policies and procedures.

In the forensic mental health setting the Department of Health (2010), based on prior work by Adshead (2004), distinguished between three types of security: physical security, procedural security and relational security. The first two are directly concerned with the technical aspects of physical safety, structural containment, the mechanisms of monitoring and surveillance (physical security) and the rational procedures that support them (procedural security); whereas relational security was described in terms of the culture of the environment, the attitudes underpinning it and the emotional qualities of the relatedness of relationships within it. To paraphrase Bion, we might also think of it as 'a planned endeavour to develop the group forces that lead to smoothly running co-operative activity [that] turn on the acquisition of knowledge and experience of the factors which make for a good group spirit' (Bion 1961, p.11).

In promoting this approach to relational security, the Department of Health is implicitly critical of systems that rely too heavily on a technical-rational approach. This opens up the potential for forms of defensive practice to emerge in an attempt to fill a theory-practice gap between what the team says it does, which Argyris and Schön (1974) refer to as its 'espoused theory', and what it actually does, which they call its 'theory-in-use'. When things go wrong in such an environment (as they inevitably will), a blame culture thrives in which personified individuals or specific sub-groups of staff – usually those closest to the patients – are blamed by those furthest away: often those who, in their failure to fully understand the importance of relational security, have set unrealistic technical-rational objectives in the first place (Rustin 2004; Cooper and Lousada 2005; see also Chapters 4, 8 and 9).

A crucial challenge is therefore to consider to what extent the work of an effective team is rooted in an informed application of pre-ordained 'treatment' regimes and the policy and procedures that support them; and to what extent it is an inter-subjective discourse, within which physical and procedural security is useful only insofar as these concepts are fully integrated into a collaborative appreciation of the 'relational security' of the team-as-a-whole: a process which Schön (1983, p.68) called 'reflection-in-action'. Two assumptions therefore underpin this chapter. The first is that 'managing the business' (including the delivery of formal therapies regimes) and 'learning how to learn from each other', though systemically related, are distinct activities that utilise distinct ways of knowing: they therefore need to be developed through different types of conversation in different spaces and places. Second, the mechanisms through which practitioners learn from participation in a culture of enquiry in the therapeutic milieu is the most neglected area of study. It is to discussion of these issues that I now turn.

REFLECTION-ON-ACTION AND REFLECTION-IN-ACTION COMPARED: THE PSYCHO-SOCIO-EDUCATIONAL DYNAMICS OF TEAM DEVELOPMENT

Schön (1987) suggests that thinking together in, and about, practice has two distinct aspects: 'reflection-in-action', discussed above, and a lower order set of skills that he calls 'reflection-on-action'. Reflection-on-action, through which practitioners learn skills from re-calling past actions and/or preparing for future action, has been extensively researched under the rubric of 'experiential learning' and has been applied to a wide range of interpersonal skills learning programmes (Kolb and Fry 1975; Boud, Keogh and Walker 1985; Heron 1992 *inter alia*). Typically this reflection-on-action involves the building of a shared team narrative of the work. These narratives will involve discussions of heroes and villains; the weak and the strong; victims, perpetrators, rescuers and bystanders; discussion of 'critical incidents' as well as discussion of the everyday practicalities pertaining directly and indirectly to aspects of 'physical' and 'procedural' dynamics outlined above. As we also know, patients disclose different aspects of their fragmented and split narratives to the responsible medical officer, the social worker, the nurse in charge and the support staff – all of which are important and necessary to understand in order to formulate a more integrated picture of the patients' broken narratives. For these reasons it is also very important that all members of the team regularly attend the team development meeting.

Whilst there is little doubt that this 'reflection-on-action' is necessary in encouraging active participation in the building of this shared narrative and for co-operative problem solving, it is suggested that for 'team development' this approach is limited because it insufficiently takes into account the social defence mechanisms and team dynamics problems that are (dis)played out in the unconscious life of the team. As such, these 'discussions' will inevitably rely upon practitioners' discussion of their 'espoused theory' rather than their deeper relational and culturally embedded 'theory in use'. Elsewhere (Scanlon 2002) I have suggested a forensic analogy, according to which this difference can be likened to those who might attempt to study the essence of a butterfly by killing it and pinning its body to a board and those who attempt to observe living butterflies as they flutter by in carefully constructed butterfly houses. The challenge for the TDC, therefore, is how to create a metaphorical butterfly house within which it is possible to reflect-in-action on the clinical material, transferred from the therapeutic milieu, into the dynamic matrices of the team development group itself.[2]

SYSTEMS, SUB-GROUPS AND PARALLEL PROCESSES

To see a world in a grain of sand,
And a heaven in a wild flower,
Hold infinity in the palm of your hand,
And eternity in an hour

Auguries of Innocence, William Blake (circa 1863)

In any system of interrelating there is an isomorphic resonance within and across the different levels and sub-groups of this system (Skynner 1989). This means that, for better and for worse, changes in any of these levels or sub-groups necessarily involve change in all the other levels and sub-systems. Within forensic systems of care the different levels and sub-systems are represented and (dis)played out between organisational, managerial, staff team and patient levels and the sub-systems within them, as well as in relation to the demands placed upon them by the wider social context (see Chapter 13). In so far as these levels and sub-systems also share a reflective space in individual members' traumatised-organisation-in-the-mind, so any change in his/her reflective capacity in one place will have an effect in all of the other places that s/he is minded to be. In the 'Systems Centred Approach' (Agazarian 1997) it is further suggested that it is more helpful to think of the basic functional unit of study in any social systems as the sub-group, the smallest functional unit of which is the pair. In other words, the only way to consider the anxiety of any individual member is to locate it in the context of his/her identification with the members of this or that sub-group.

---

2   This analogy may be particularly apt given that the etymology of 'psyche' refers both to 'mind/soul' and to 'butterfly'.

Membership of sub-groups is both formally defined, for example in terms of occupational group, gender, age and ethnicity, and also in terms of more abstract connections such as the shared expression of grievance, love, hatred, desire and so on. In this sense the sub-groups are always fluid. Sometimes a staff member might find themself aligned with a colleague (or patient) in one or other sub-grouping; at other times, in opposition. The individual staff member might also find themself in an oppositional sub-group that is identified with the real and imagined concerns of the Ministry of Justice, the patients' victims or the general public – for example, in identification with a wish to punish or vilify. In this sense the relationships within and between traumatised-organisations-in-the-minds and their institutional and social contexts are complex and highly stressful.

A number of theorists have suggested a further reflective aspect of these isomorphic resonances with reference to both a clinical and educational application of the concept of 'parallel process'. In its clinical application this concept has recently been described as 'offence paralleling' behaviour (Daffern *et al.* 2010) – although a shared understanding of the ways in which patients' disturbance has been enacted in the therapeutic milieu has long been a tradition in the Therapeutic Communities movement (Jones 1968; Main 1983; Norton 1992; Whitely 1986 *inter alia*). It is beyond the scope of this chapter to rehearse this theory in detail. However, put simply, 'offence paralleling' is an approach to risk assessment and intervention that emerges out of careful observations and analyses of the ways in which patients' deeply engrained maladaptive relational patterns, often born of early traumatic experience and enacted in their offending behaviour, are unconsciously transferred into and played out in the here-and-now of the institutional setting. It is both a communication of the patients' early traumatisation and an expression of their 'criminogenic needs' (see Chapter 6). As an adjunct to an effective intervention strategy, the institutional response to these 'offence paralleling' enactments is crucial in determining outcome. At its most helpful, the institutional response, rooted in careful examination of the teams' reactions, enables a reflective understanding of the communicative and expressive aspects of these enactments in ways that challenge rather than gratify them (Norton and Dolan 1995; Shine and Morris 2000). To be able to do this effectively, the team must have the reflective spaces and places available to think about the ways in which the parallel processes that had their origins in the patients' early history and offending are transferred from the there-and-then of the clinical context into the here-and-now of the Team Development group, making the dynamics available for the type of enquiry that is reflection-in-action. When this works well, it is as if the network of communications that is (dis)played out in all the different levels and sub-groups within the therapeutic milieu is resonating on the same frequency. By analogy with the therapeutic task, the educational task of the team development group is to enable an exchange and translation of these different narratives into an ever more articulate understanding of the 'personal, interpersonal and inter-system problems…of impulses, defences and relations as these are expressed and arranged socially' (Main 1983).

At this point it does not matter whether the team begins by talking about the patients or their own worries, because each level and every sub-group in the system contains, and is contained by, all the others. In this context the team development group, as *reflective practicum* (Schön 1983), becomes a 'transitional and intermediate space' relatively free from the pressures of the 'real world' of practice, within which the dynamics of the traumatised-organisation-in-the-mind can be safely explored and thought about. With skilled facilitation, this reflective space can then become an associative world of imagination in which all the members reflect, and reflect upon, what they and their patients have been doing together. Just as the team is expected to become the archivist of the therapeutic narrative, so too the Team Development group – including the TDC – becomes the archive-and-archivists of the more unconscious narratives that are expressed in these parallel processes. Elsewhere (Scanlon 1997) I have suggested that there is much to be learned from these associative and imaginative conversations, providing that all remain aware that what they are individually or collectively imagining is not 'the truth' but a situated rendering of a different set of invested narratives: formulations to be further discussed, refined or dismissed as these reflective conversations unfold.

Thus, a major difference between reflection-on-action and reflection-in-action is a spatio-temporal one, in that the latter is concerned with getting at the knowledge that is unconsciously embedded in the 'here-and-now' of the team dynamic, whereas the former is primarily concerned with reflecting on the 'there-and-then' of previous, or future, encounters. A central task for the TDC is to optimise a facilitating environment (Carlyle and Evans 2005; Hinshelwood 1994; James 1994) within which conversations can move between the 'figure' and 'ground' of reflection-on-action and reflection-in-action: between narrative discussion of consciously lived experience and the unconscious impact of the dynamics as they are played out in these parallel processes. The challenge for the TDC, as for all good educators, is to establish what is already known and to facilitate learning accordingly (Jarvis 1987; Knowles 1980). S/he may want to encourage the sort of reflection-on-action that would focus on the manifest content of the work, in ways that would allow the emergent narratives and the rhythms of the clinical encounters to be more closely observed and so enable practitioners to get to know each other better. When a team is more cohesive and more willing and better able to think together, the TDC might want to encourage a more free-floating conversation that enables the sort of imaginative associations that would allow the tacitly contained material to emerge in the parallel processes. The TDC would also need to be aware that to encourage this more associative style of presentation might run the risk of the discussion becoming so divergent and fragmented that the primary work task may become obscured, lost or avoided. Indeed, Schön (1987, p.60) suggests that because reflection-in-action relies on these more associative responses, there is a danger that the team members can sometimes become so convinced of their own 'healing powers' that a defensive complacency may set in, within which its members become closed-minded and no longer feel the need to reflect deeply upon what they are doing together. One tell-tale sign that these dynamics may be at work is when a team member (usually a 'senior' member) imagines that they can offer this type of consultancy to their own team or when a team colludes with an idea that they do not need an external perspective and can operate as a peer-group. In my view the former is completely impossible and whilst the latter, the peer-group, may be possible in principle, it is often so difficult to 'see the wood for the trees' that I could not recommend it. One of the critical skills of the TDC, therefore, is to be a highly (re)active and versatile mediator of and moderator for these associative processes, in ways that will both support and challenge team members to think together about the complex (dis)organisational dynamics at the heart of the work.

It will also be clear that these complex reciprocal processes are not linear but (re)iterative and that even the most cohesive team may sometimes need to be directed towards more focused reflection-on-action. For example, following a serious incident it may be necessary to return to a more detailed examination of the actual text and/or context of the event to allow for the type of critical incident analysis which, while of limited value as a stand-alone intervention, does enable a more cohesive team to work through the incident rather than becoming stuck or traumatised in relation to it. Similarly, a skilfully directed rehearsal about how to make a particularly difficult challenge to patient(s) or colleagues, or feeding back to 'the management' on behalf of the system-as-a-whole, may allow the team to be better prepared to do this more effectively and more constructively.

CONCLUDING REMARKS

The aim of this chapter has been to describe the ways in which 'relational security' can be optimised by enabling practitioners in forensic settings to take up membership of their role in the team. My argument has been that, construed in these ways, relational security is very little to do with mandatory training or with individual staff members developing a technical competence in this or that treatment modality but is much more about a readiness to join and actively participate in reflective interpersonal, and inter-professional, conversations within a wider culture of enquiry. This, of course, raises serious questions about the strategic implementation of such team-focused interventions including specific training implications, clear job descriptions and person specifications for those who are charged with offering this type of intervention. By extension this approach also has clear implications for more inter-professional education in the basic training of all mental health, social care and community justice practitioners in order to prepare them better for the challenge of more effective collaborative working (World Health Organisation 2010). My plea is to join with others to invite further inter-professional and collaborative research into this much-neglected area of work.

ACKNOWLEDGEMENTS

I would like to acknowledge Ros Abbott, John Adlam, Godfried Attafua, Jo-anne Carlyle and Ian Simpson with whom I work in the 'Reflective Practice Team Development' project in South London and Maudsley Foundation NHS Trust and/or 'The Station' and/or SAM Training and Consultancy. I would also particularly like to acknowledge my indebtedness to my friends and colleagues David Armstrong, Tavistock Consultancy Services and Dr Earl Hopper from whom I have learned enormously. Finally I would like to express my hope for a day when we can all feel proud of what we have learned together.

REFERENCES

Adshead, G. (1991) 'The forensic psychotherapist: dying breed or evolving species?' *Psychiatric Bulletin 15*, 410-412.

Adshead, G. (2004) 'Three Degrees of Security: Attachment and Forensic Institutions.' In F. Pfäfflin and G. Adshead (eds) *A Matter of Security: The Application of Attachment Theory to Forensic Psychiatry and Psychotherapy.* London: Jessica Kingsley Publishers.

Agazarian, Y. (1997) *Systems-Centered Therapy for Groups.* New York: Guildford Press.

Aiyegbusi, A. and Clarke, J. (eds) (2008) *Relationships with Offenders: An Introduction to the Psychodynamics of Forensic Mental Health Nursing.* London: Jessica Kingsley Publishers.

Aiyegbusi, A. and Kelly, G. (eds) (2012, forthcoming) *Professional and Therapeutic Boundaries in Forensic Mental Health.* London: Jessica Kingsley Publishers.

Argyris, C. and Schön, D. (1974) *Theory in Practice: Increasing Professional Effectiveness.* San Francisco: Jossey Bass.

Armstrong, D. (2005) *Organization in the Mind: Psychoanalysis, Group Relations and Organizational Consultancy.* London: Karnac.

Arnold, M. (2004) *The Collected Poems of Matthew Arnold.* London: Kessinger.

Ballat, J. and Campling, P. (2011) *Intelligent Kindness: Reforming the Culture of Healthcare.* Glasgow: Royal College of Psychiatrists.

Boud, D., Keogh, R. and Walker, D. (1985) *Reflection: Turning Experience into Learning.* London: Kogan Page.

Bevington, D. and Fuggle, P. (2012) 'Supporting and Enhancing Mentalization in Community Outreach Teams Working with "Hard-to-Reach" Youth: The AMBIT Approach.' In N. Midgley and I. Vrouvra (eds) *Minding the Child: Mentalization-Based Treatment for Children, Young People and Families.* London: Routledge.

Bion, W.R. (1961) *Experiences in Groups.* London: Tavistock.

Bion, W.R. (1970) *Attention and Interpretation.* London: Tavistock.

Bion, W.R. (1975) *Brazilian Lectures.* Rio de Janeiro: Imago editorial.

Blumenthal, S., Ruszczynski, S., Richards, R. and Brown, M. (2011) 'Evaluation of the impact of a consultation in a secure setting.' *Criminal Behaviour and Mental Health 21*, 233–244.

Bramley, W. (1990) 'Staff Sensitivity Groups: a conductor's field experiences.' *Group Analysis 23*, 301–316.

Campling, P., Davies, S. and Farquharson, G. (2004) (eds) *From Toxic Institutions to Therapeutic Environments: Residential Settings in Mental Health Services.* London: Gaskell Publishers.

Canning, J. and Babb, R. (2010) Interface of Meaning and Projection Formulation (IMPF). Millfields Unit, John Howard Centre (personal communication).

Carlyle, J. and Evans, C. (2005). 'Containing containers: attention to the 'innerface' and 'outerface' of groups in secure institutions.' *Group Analysis 38*, 3, 395–408.

Coltart, N. (1993) *Slouching towards Bethlehem: And Further Psychoanalytic Explorations.* London: Free Association Books.

Cooper, A. and Lousada, J. (2005) *Borderline Welfare: Feeling and Fear of Feeling in Modern Welfare.* London: Karnac.

Cordess, C. and Cox, M. (1996) *Forensic Psychotherapy: Crime, Psychodynamics and the Offender Patient.* London: Jessica Kingsley Publishers.

Cordess, C., Welldon, E. and Riley, W. (1994) 'Psychodynamic forensic psychotherapy: An account of a day-release course.' *Psychiatric Bulletin 18*, 88–90.

Daffern, M., Lawrence, Jones, L. and Shine, J. (2010) *Offence Paralleling Behaviour: A Case Formulation Approach to Offender Assessment and Intervention.* Chichester: John Wiley.

Dartington, T. (2010) *Managing Vulnerability: The Underlying Dynamics of Systems of Care.* London: Karnac.

Department for Communities and Local Government (2010) *Meeting the psychological and emotional needs of homeless people: Non-statutory guidance on dealing with complex psychological and emotional needs.* HMSO: Department for Communities and Local Government.

Department of Health (2010) *'See, Think, Act': Your Guide to Relational Security.* HMSO: Department of Health.

Freud, S. (1937) *Analysis Terminable and Interminable.* Standard Edition Volume 23.

Gabbard, G.O. and Wilkinson, S. (1994). *Management of Counter-transference with Borderline Patients.* Washington, DC: American Psychiatric Press.

Gordon, J. and Kirtchuk, G. (2008) (eds) *Psychic Assaults and Frightened Clinicians: Countertransference in Forensic Settings.* London: Karnac.

Haigh, R. (2000) 'Support systems. 2. Staff sensitivity groups.' *Advances in Psychiatric Treatment 6*, 312–319.

Hartley, P. and Kennard, D. (2009) (eds) *Staff Support Groups In The Helping Professions. Principles and Pitfalls.* London and New York: Routledge.

Heron, J. (1992) *Feeling and Personhood. Psychology in Another Key.* London: Sage.

Hinshelwood, R.D. (1994) 'Attacks on the Reflective Space.' In M. Pines and V.L. Schermer (eds) *Ring of Fire.* London: Routledge.

Hoggett, P. (2005) 'A Service to the Public: The Containment of Ethical and Moral Conflict by Public Bureaucracies.' In P. duGay (ed.) *The Values of Bureaucracy.* Oxford: Oxford University Press.

Honig, B. (1996) 'Difference, Dilemmas and the Politics of Home.' In S. Benhabib (ed.) *Democracy and Difference: Contesting the Boundaries of the Political.* Princeton: Princeton University Press.

Hopper, E. (2003) *Traumatic Experience in the Unconscious Life of Groups: The Fourth Basic Assumption: Incohesion: Aggregation/Massification or (ba) I:A/M.* London: Jessica Kingsley Publishers.

Hopper, E. (2011) *Trauma in Organisations.* London: Karnac.

James, D. (1994) 'Holding and Containing in the Group and in Society.' In D. Brown and L. Zinkin (eds) *The Psyche and the Social World. Developments in Group-Analytic Theory.* London: Routledge.

Jarvis, P. (1987) *Adult Learning in the Social Context.* London: Croom Helm.

Johnson, R. and Haigh, R. (2010) 'Social psychiatry and social policy for the 21st century – new concepts for new needs: the "psychologically-informed environment".' *Mental Health and Social Inclusion 14*, 4, 30–35.

Johnson, R. and Haigh, R. (2011) 'Social psychiatry and social policy for the 21st century – new concepts for new needs: the "Enabling Environments" initiative.' *Mental Health and Social Inclusion 15*, 1, 17–26.

Jones, M. (1968) *Social Psychiatry in Practice: The Idea of the Therapeutic Community.* Harmondsworth: Penguin.

Kanas, N. (1986) 'Support groups for mental health staff.' *International Journal of Group Psychotherapy 36*, 279–296.

Knowles, M. (1980) *The Modern Practice of Adult Education: From Pedagogy to Androgogy.* Englewood, New Jersey: Prentice-Hall.

Kolb, D.A. and Fry, R. (1975) 'Towards an applied theory of Experiential Learning.' In C. Cooper (ed.) *The Theories of Group Process.* London: John Wiley.

Mace, C. (2007) 'Mindfulness in psychotherapy: an introduction.' *Advances in Psychiatric Treatment 13*, 147–154.

Main, T.F. (1983) *The Ailment and Other Essays.* London: Free Association Books.

McGauley, G. (2002) 'Forensic psychotherapy in secure settings.' *Journal of Forensic Psychiatry 13*, 9–13.

Menzies-Lyth, I. (1992) *Containing Anxiety in Institutions. Selected Essays (Vol 1).* London: Free Association Books.

Norton, K. (1992) 'A culture of enquiry: its preservation or loss.' *Therapeutic Communities 13*, 3–25.

Norton, K. and Dolan, B. (1995) 'Acting-out and the Institutional Response.' *Journal of Forensic Psychiatry 6*, 2, 317–332.

Norton, K. and McGauley, G. (2000) 'Forensic psychotherapy in Britain: its role in assessment, treatment and training.' *Criminal Behaviour and Mental Health 10*, S82–S90.

Novakovic, A. (2002) 'Work with psychotic patients in a Rehabilitation Unit: a short term staff support group with a nursing team.' *Group Analysis 35*, 560.

Obholzer, A and V.Z. Roberts (eds) (1994) *The Unconscious at Work: Individual and Organizational Stress in the Human Services.* London: Routledge.

Pietroni, P.C. (1992) 'Towards reflective practice – the languages of health and social care.' *Journal of International Care 6*, 1, 7–16.

Reiss, D. and Kirtchuk, G. (2009). 'Interpersonal dynamics and multidisciplinary team work.' *Advances in Psychiatric Treatment 15*, 462–469.

Roberts, V.Z. (1994) 'The Self-appointed Impossible Task'. In A. Obholzer and V.Z. Roberts (eds) *The Unconscious at Work: Individual and Organizational Stress in the Human Services*. London: Routledge.

Royal College of Psychiatrists (2010) 'Enabling Environments.' Available at www.rcpsych.ac.uk/quality/quality,accreditationaudit/enablingenvironments.aspx, accessed on 24 January 2012.

Rustin, M. (2004) 'Re-thinking Audit and Inspection.' *Soundings 64*, 86–107.

Ruszczynski, S. (2008) 'Thoughts from Consulting in Secure Settings: do Forensic Institutions need Psychotherapy?' In J. Gordon and G. Kirtchuk (eds) *Psychic Assaults and Frightened Clinicians: Countertransference in Forensic Settings*. London: Karnac.

Ryle, G. (1949) *The Concept of Mind*. London: Hutchinson.

Scanlon, C. (2002) 'Group supervision of individual cases in the training of psychodynamic practitioners: towards a group-analytic model?' *British Journal of Psychotherapy 19*, 2, 219–235.

Scanlon, C. and Adlam, J. (2011a) '"Who watches the watchers?" Observing the dangerous liaisons between forensic patients and their carers in the perverse panopticon.' *Organisational and Social Dynamics 11*, 2, 175–195.

Scanlon, C. and Adlam, J. (2011b) 'Disorganised Responses to Refusal and Spoiling in Traumatised Organisations.' In E. Hopper (ed) *Trauma and Organisations*. London: Karnac.

Schön, D.A. (1983) *The Reflective Practitioner*. New York: Basic Books.

Schön, D.A. (1987) *Educating the Reflective Practitioner*. New York: Basic Books.

Shine, J. and Morris, M. (2000) 'Addressing criminogenic needs in a prison therapeutic community.' *Therapeutic Communities 21*, 3, 197–219.

Simpson, I. (2010) 'Containing the Uncontainable: A Role for Staff Support Groups.' In J. Radcliffe., K. Hajek, J. Carson and O. Manor (eds) *Psychological Groupwork with Acute Psychiatric Inpatients*. London: Whiting and Birch.

Skynner, A.C.R. (1989) *Institutes and How to Survive Them: Mental Health Training and Consultation*. London: Routledge.

Thorndycraft, B. and McCabe, J. (2008) 'The challenge of working with staff groups in the caring professions: the importance of the "team development and reflective practice group".' *British Journal of Psychotherapy 24*, 2, 167–183.

Whiteley, J.S. (1986) 'Sociotherapy and Psychotherapy in the treatment of personality disorder: a discussion paper.' *Journal of the Royal Society of Medicine 79*, 721–725.

World Health Organisation (2010) *Framework for Action on Interprofessional Education & Collaborative Practice*. Geneva: WHO.

Chapter 15

SOME CHALLENGES TO THE CAPACITY TO THINK, LINK AND HOPE IN THE PROVISION OF PSYCHOTHERAPY FOR THE LEARNING DISABLED[1]

Earl Hopper

Earl Hopper closes this volume with his description of the challenges to the capacity to think, link and hope that are associated with the provision of psychotherapy for the learning disabled. Echoing the earlier chapters by Corbett and Sinason, he shows how this entails working in a society that devalues the unintelligent and highly disabled and diminishes those who work with them as 'nice' and 'caring' but incapable of understanding the complex internal worlds of forensic patients. He describes the strain of those who work with such patients and cautions against burnout. Hopper joins with Ruszczynski and Scanlon in stressing the importance of supervision, consultation and team meetings for open and honest discussion of the work, suggesting that working within organisations presents its own problems, although it is virtually inevitable that the provision of psychotherapy for the learning disabled will be within organisational contexts. He expresses his curiosity about what draws us to this work and describes his own motivation. His comments have profound implications for all practitioners within the forensic field.

---

1   I am indebted to Al Corbett for the title of this presentation, which is, in effect, an attempt to answer a question that he asked me: what are some of the challenges to the capacity to think, link and hope in forensic settings in which psychotherapy is provided for the learning disabled? I have been inspired by the work of Walter Stone (1998) with the chronically mentally ill, and by the work of Frances Tustin (1972) with autistic children and with autistic anxieties in general. I have been asked to focus on my own work, and, therefore, I have not attempted to review the literature, although extensive bibliography is provided in the publications cited.

In this chapter I will discuss some of the challenges to our capacity to think, link and hope that are associated with the provision of psychotherapy for the learning disabled. This discussion is based on my experience as a supervisor and as a consultant to organisations in which such services are provided. Given how difficult and dispiriting this work can be, I am curious about what draws us to it. I will also offer some suggestions about meeting the challenges to a professional frame of mind as best we can.

Assuming that we agree on the meaning of 'thinking' and 'linking', I would define 'hope', in the context of a secular orientation, as the ability and willingness to exercise the transcendent imagination, that is, to imagine how things might be better and how we might make them better. I am not referring to infantile, pie in the sky hope, but to mature hope, which is a virtue and a developmental achievement (Hopper 2003a, 2009). Hope is always a function of making connections, both intra-personally and inter-personally, within a particular social, cultural and political context (Hopper 2011).

I will consider some of the challenges to our capacity to think, link and hope in providing psychotherapy for the learning disabled in terms of our society, profession, patients and unconscious group dynamics associated with traumatic experience, as well as our own personalities and conflicts, in order:

1. Among the challenges that emanate from our society, I would emphasise the devaluation of the unintelligent and highly dependent, and, therefore, of those of us in the helping professions associated with them. These attitudes are embedded in the cultures of most societies (Corbett 2010). England is hardly unusual in harbouring such views.

    Consider the current, ferocious cutbacks by government agencies of various services for the learning disabled and of financial subsidies for the provision of them. This is not merely a matter of reducing public expenditure, but also of a heightened sense that the learning disabled do not and cannot contribute to the economic well-being of the society, and, therefore, do not *deserve* these services and financial subsidies. Ironically, these 'cutbacks' only make the problem of how to look after the learning disabled much worse and more visible, leading to more extreme solutions.

The most extreme forms of devaluation of the learning disabled have involved attempts to rid societies of them by purifying the gene pool. Having first been defined as rubbish and outside the moral community, they were castrated, as well as asphyxiated and burned. This depended on the development of an ideology of extreme rationality that defined human beings as material objects in the context of economic and industrial efficiency, combined with the development of political romanticism, as occurred, for example, in Nazi Germany. It is interesting that the practice of eugenics continued even after World War II in various so-called 'enlightened' countries, and that in the politics of various kinds of final solutions knowledge of genetic mutation was disavowed.

Less extreme forms of the devaluation of the learning disabled are manifest in the fact that those who are employed to help them have tended to be women and immigrants who lack higher education and marketable skills, and who must accept what work is available to them. Their work reconfirms their low status, and their low status reconfirms the low value given to such work.

Societal devaluation can also be seen in the tendency for residential care facilities to be located far away from the original homes of the residents. In part this may be a matter of the availability of large, relatively inexpensive buildings and the ready supply of relatively inexpensive labour, but it is also a wish to keep the learning disabled out of sight, perhaps especially those with Down's syndrome. (This makes it difficult for the families of a learning disabled child to provide even absentee parenting.)

2. Differentiating societal challenges from those that emanate from a specific profession is difficult. However, our colleagues are used as containers for projections of feelings of helplessness, despair and vulnerability. These projections emanate not only from their patients and the families of their patients, but also from people and institutions associated with the field of learning disability. For example, our colleagues are in continuous struggle with powerful governmental and charitable agencies for financial aid and general support, and they often function as spokespersons for their patients and clients who lack their own 'voices'. In this

context, our colleagues are regarded as lacking in the capacity to be rational, and to make tough choices. They are regarded as excessively demanding and overly identified with the learning disabled.

Many psychiatrists, psychoanalysts and group analysts tend to regard those who work in the field of learning disability as 'nice' and 'caring' but incapable of understanding the complex internal worlds of forensic patients. These patients are often devious with respect to their internal objects and people in authority in their external worlds. It is difficult not to collude with such projections. Thus, therapists and counsellors in this sub-profession tend to devalue themselves in comparison with those in the higher echelons of psychiatry, psychoanalysis and group analysis, who are regarded as excessively 'intellectual' and 'elitist'. This splitting between the overvaluation of the paternal principles of 'theoretical understanding' and the undervaluation of the maternal principles of 'helping' fails to appreciate the essential value of kindness and compassion. Theoretical understanding without empathy provides little help for any kind of patient, learning disabled or otherwise.

Our colleagues do not always get much gratification from their limited clinical 'achievements'. Although it is marvellous when a learning disabled patient has a breakthrough in, for example, his capacity to reflect upon his actions and gain some sense of having a mind of his own, this is often a consolation prize. In comparison to the presentations of certain kinds of psychoanalysts, which often begin with a few lines about their clients being highly intelligent, we cannot present our cases by saying, 'Of course, he is highly stupid, in fact as thick as two planks'. In other words, we cannot identify with the brilliant. We must find other sources of gratification in our work. (Actually, what is the point of saying that a patient is highly intelligent? To illustrate that the patient is unable to realise his potential? Or to convey that the patient is unable to use our brilliant interpretations?)

3. Many challenges to our capacity to think, link and hope emanate from our learning disabled patients themselves. They really do need us as auxiliary egos to help them name feelings and ideas, and to have a sense of their own location in time and space.

This puts a constant strain on our patience and commitment to the work. Many of our colleagues have little respite from their chronic sense of guilt that they are not doing enough to make things better for their patients. They also tend to experience something akin to post-natal depression, based on the mother's envy of the infant who is regarded as having a legitimate right to make extreme demands on her ability and willingness to provide the extra care on which the infant's survival depends.

The ability to sustain mature hope requires the ability to recognise changes both in environment and in moods as well as in levels of achievement with respect to various goals. However, in our learning disabled patients such changes are limited, and even these changes take a very long time. Moreover, the learning disabled are usually not sufficiently self-reflective to know when such changes have occurred.

In this context, consider what Durkheim (1951) called 'fatalistic suicide' (which he did not really discuss in his great book *Suicide*, but only mentioned in a footnote). Durkheim thought that fatalistic suicide was over-represented among slaves and other captive people whose lives would never improve. They could not imagine that things would or could ever get better. For example, fatalistic suicide would be over-represented among the captives in death camps, as seen in the so-called 'Muselmen' who were identified more in terms of their loss of hope than their loss of nourishment and physical well-being. In my view fatalistic suicide not only occurs among people whose resources are very limited, but also among those who perceive that reality is, and will forever be, unchanging: never getting better and never getting worse. This is likely to be even more debilitating than the experience of a fixed level of deprivation, because it is likely to lead to paralysis of the ability and willingness to imagine that life can be better. This reminds me of Winnicott's (1949) discussion of birth trauma and feelings of helplessness in which he refers to 'the intolerable nature of experiencing something without any knowledge of when it will end', as in the case of 'a prisoner of war' (1949, p.184).

The paralysis of imagination that life can be better permeates the lives of the learning disabled. It also permeates our therapeutic relationships with them, no matter how hard we try to focus on what might be possible for them. To acknowledge that our work involves something like watching paint dry is difficult. It can be dispiriting and demoralising. Burn-out is commonplace. If the truth be known, we often ask ourselves 'Why bother?' There are no easy answers to such a question, but it is important to recognise that even asking it is a kind of act of fatalistic suicide.

It is also important to recognise that learning disabled patients tend to have been traumatised, both as a result of the vicissitudes of their learning disability and the responses of other people to this, and in terms of their inability to understand and negotiate their sexual and aggressive desires and impulses. Many have been sexually abused, and many have sexually abused others. Containment and self-control is not easy for them.

The dynamics of the intrapersonal and the interpersonal lives of the traumatised must, therefore, be noted. The phenomenology of the trauma of helplessness and failed dependency in the context of the centrality of human relationships, which are at the core of the human condition, involves:

- the fear of annihilation characterised by psychotic anxieties associated with fission and fragmentation, on the one hand, and psychotic anxieties associated with fusion and confusion, on the other

- the use of disassociation, psychic retreats and encapsulations as defences against these anxieties, involving the development of autistic barriers to communication.

Such patients get under our skin, and try constantly to get under our skin, in their attempts to communicate through projective identification as a means of evacuation, control and sadistic attack. They do this especially in the service of communication via enactment, which is virtually the only way that learning disabled patients can communicate what they cannot symbolise. Such patients do this not only because of their limited capacity to conceptualise and verbalise their experience, but also because their traumatic experience has limited their capacity to symbolise. As their auxiliary egos we are especially likely to experience their autistic anxieties and defences against them. Under these conditions it is difficult to remain 'live company' (Alvarez 1992).

4. The challenges presented by unconscious group dynamics associated with traumatic experience cannot be avoided (Hopper 2012). It is well known that in response to various conditions, groups and organisations tend to regress. One of the most comprehensive explanations for such regression is offered by Bion's (1961) theory of basic assumptions, which has been developed and refined by many. In this theory the basic assumptions of pairing, fight/flight and dependency are characterised by particular sets of co-constructed roles which members of the group are prone to enact based on their particular personality characteristics. This relationship between the dynamics of the group and the dynamics of the members' personalities has been discussed in terms of valence, role suction and personification. Each basic assumption involves attacks on thinking, linking and mature hoping.

In my own work (Hopper 2003b) I have developed a theory of a fourth basic assumption, which I have called Incohesion: Aggregation/Massification or (ba) I:A/M. Incohesion is especially concerned with linking. The fourth basic assumption of Incohesion: Aggregation/Massification is typical of groups and organisations which have been traumatised and/or which are associated with traumatic experience. This may be considered in terms of strain, cumulative and/or catastrophic trauma. Their underlying common denominator is the experience of failed dependency. Patterns of aggregation are derived from the fear of annihilation as expressed in psychic fission and fragmentation; and patterns of massification are derived from the fear of annihilation as expressed in psychic fusion and confusion with others. Aggregation oscillates with massification both on the basis of these psychic polarities, and on the basis of various structural pressures and dilemmas within the structures of the social system itself, such as those associated with the causes of anomie (Hopper 1981, 2003b).

The role of the 'lone wolf observer' is typical of aggregation, and the role of 'cheerleader' is typical of massification. Those with a valence for aggregation roles tend to have alienated, schizoid and 'crustacean' characters; and those with a valence for massification roles tend to have identity seeking, merger hungry and 'amoeboid' characters. These two sets of roles also tend to suck in those people who are dominated by particular kinds of perversions and perverse character structures, aggregation roles attracting sadists, and massification roles, masochists.

Such people tend to personify processes of aggregation and processes of massification, respectively.

The dynamics of Incohesion are typical of organisations such as prisons, mental hospitals and clinics for providing care and treatment for the learning disabled (Corbett, Cottis and Lloyd 2012) and other organisations in the forensic field, in which experiences of trauma are ubiquitous. The clinical and managerial staff of such organisations are chronically exposed to the suction of roles associated with Incohesion. They are tempted to enact scenarios associated with this basic assumption. When aggregation prevails, they are tempted to destroy their own organisations while working in a 'disassociated' state of mind, characterised by ritualisation and routinisation, having lost their ability to identify with their patients. When massification prevails, they are tempted to become over-involved with their patients, attempting to compensate for the inadequate parenting that they have so often experienced. In the former case, it becomes easy to defraud the organisation, for example by 'cooking the books', as a form of compensation for the feeling that it has been necessary to give too much to the organisation, being caught up in the exigencies of fundraising and attending too many 'absolutely necessary' conferences; and in the latter case, it becomes easy to be drained of energy and vitality, and to function as a slave to the organisation. Both responses are versions of what occurs in post-natal depression, and are in essence forms of a sense of compensatory entitlement.

Many members of the sub-profession of psychotherapy for the learning disabled tend both consciously to dis-identify with their patients and unconsciously to identify with them, often simultaneously. Although they are more intelligent, competent, articulate, powerful and potent than their patients, unconsciously they have very low self-esteem, at least in my experience of my colleagues. This combination leads them simultaneously both consciously to empathise with their patients and unconsciously to distance themselves from them. They tend, therefore, simultaneously both to make links with their patients and to destroy these links. Our colleagues are hopeful for their patients, and at the same time they are pessimistic about their welfare and development. These ambivalent attitudes are often enacted in their behaviour towards their patients and colleagues. For example, when the anxieties associated with this contradiction are felt to be acute, colleagues have to cut off emotionally from their patients, becoming somewhat schizoid in their general affective response to them. Another response to these anxieties is to become masochistic in the work, also sacrificing the possibility of a satisfying and active personal life, leading to burn-out.

In the context of the dynamics of the basic assumption of Incohesion, staff of organisations in the field of learning disability also have opportunities for the realisation of their own traumatic experience. This may involve the enactment of sado-masochist fantasies and the repetition of perversions in the sense of corruption and/or turning a blind eye to theft, fraud and other kinds of criminality (turning away from the true, involving theft, fraud and other kinds of criminality). They are tempted to abide by the leaden rule of forensic psychotherapy: 'Do unto others as you have been done by.' In fact, in the last few months the mass media in Britain has carried reports about staff in care homes for the learning disabled who allegedly committed fraud in connection with applications for grants from charities. The painful and terrifying reports of alleged abuse of the aged learning disabled residents of care homes offer an extreme case of what we must be careful to understand in order to be able to avoid.

There are, in contrast, more 'positive' reasons for coming into this branch of the profession. I would describe my own motivation for coming into the field primarily in terms of working through my own need to make reparation, to seek forgiveness, and to make sense of my own traumatic experience and that of people who are close to me. This involves trying to stay in touch with parts of myself that I would rather repress and disavow, the integration of which is a matter of my own personal growth. It is important to me to honour the values of psychoanalysis and group analysis, which are associated with healing in the sense of making whole rather than of 'curing' or 'treating' (Pines 1998).

Many of us are motivated to facilitate the healing process, in the best sense of the notion of facilitating, as a task of 'organic gardening', based on respect for the possibilities of natural growth in conditions of safety. This is a matter of being able and willing to understand transference and countertransference processes in the search for truthful insight, and to avoid the temptations of enactment, which is entirely possible in psychotherapy for the learning disabled, as it is in psychotherapy in general.

It is particularly important to try to avoid burn-out and recognise the warning signals. It is necessary to refuse to romanticise suffering and to succumb to the temptations of fatalistic suicide, which merge into the temptations of altruistic homicide. Our colleagues who provide psychotherapy for the learning disabled need a bit of slack, they need time and space to look after themselves. It is essential to provide opportunities for supervision and consultation in which transference and countertransference processes can be understood and worked through. Psychotherapy for the learning disabled stirs up primitive emotions and impulses which may be unconscious as well as defying intellectual understanding.

Group supervision and consultation contribute to the building up of cultures that support the best features of our work. Colleagues are tolerant of each other and are able to support each other. The strengths and weaknesses of their work should not be encapsulated in supervisory dyads. Group supervision also maximises the professional development of the supervisors who are rarely able to carry the full emotional weight of supervisory transference and countertransference processes on their own (see Chapter 14).

It is vital for us to look after our organisations, which in turn will look after us. In practice this means team meetings in which open and honest discussion of all aspects of our work can occur. Such meetings are essential for the health and well-being of our organisations in the context of which psychotherapy for the learning disabled is provided. With insight and mutual support, the enactment of our own psycho-social dynamics can be in the service of good organisational citizenship (Hopper 2012).

REFERENCES

Alvarez, A. (1992) *Live Company.* London and New York: Tavistock/Routledge.

Bion, W.R. (1961) *Experiences in Groups and Other Papers.* London: Tavistock.

Corbett, A. (2010) 'The Weakest Link: the Social Unconscious and its impact on an analytic group for offenders with intellectual disabilities.' Unpublished paper.

Corbett, A, Cottis, T. and Lloyd, E. (2012) 'The Survival and Development of a Traumatised Clinic for Psychotherapy for People with Intellectual Disabilities.' In E. Hopper (ed.) (2012) *Trauma and Organisations.* London: Karnac.

Durkheim, E. (1951) *Suicide.* Glencoe, Illinois: The Free Press.

Hopper, E. (1981) *Social Mobility: A Study of Social Control and Insatiability.* Oxford: Blackwell.

Hopper, E. (2003a) 'On the Nature of Hope in Psychoanalysis and Group Analysis.' In *The Social Unconscious: Selected Papers.* London: Jessica Kingsley Publishers.

Hopper, E. (2003b) *Traumatic Experience in the Unconscious Life of Groups.* London: Jessica Kingsley Publishers.

Hopper, E. (2009) 'Building bridges between psychoanalysis and group analysis in theory and clinical practice.' *Group Analysis 42*, 4, 406–425.

Hopper, E. (ed.) (2012) *Trauma and Organisations*. London: Karnac Books.

Hopper, E. and Weinberg, H. (eds) (2011) *The Social Unconscious in Persons, Groups and Societies, Volume I: Mainly Theory*. London: Karnac Books.

Pines, M. (1998) 'Group Analysis and Healing.' In *Circular Reflections: Selected Papers on Group Analysis and Psychoanalysis*. London: Jessica Kingsley Publishers.

Stone, W. (1998) 'Affect and Therapeutic Process in Groups for Chronically Mentally Ill Persons.' *Journal of Psychotherapy Practice and Research 7*, 208–216. Reprinted in 2009 in W. Stone (ed.) *Contributions of Self Psychology to Group Psychotherapy: Selected Papers*. London: Karnac Books.

Tustin, F. (1972) *Autism and Childhood Psychosis*. London: Hogarth Press.

Winnicott, D.W. (1949) 'Birth Memories, Birth Trauma and Anxieties.' In *Collected Papers: Through Paediatrics to Psychoanalysis*. London: Tavistock Publishers.

LIST OF CONTRIBUTORS

John Adlam is Consultant Adult Psychotherapist in Reflective Practice and Team Development for forensic secure services in South London and Maudsley Foundation NHS Trust and he is also Principal Adult Psychotherapist and Lead for Group Psychotherapies at the South West London and St George's Adult Eating Disorders Service. He trained in Psychoanalytical Group Psychotherapy at the Tavistock Centre and in Forensic Psychotherapeutic Studies at the Portman Clinic. He is a member of the Psycho-Social Studies Network Steering Group, a member of the Faculty for Homeless Health and an Associate Editor of the journal *Free Associations*. Together with Christopher Scanlon he has published widely in the fields of psychosocial approaches to personality disorder, homelessness, dangerousness and social exclusion. He has been a Visiting Lecturer in Forensic Mental Health at St George's University of London and at the Portman Clinic and was formerly Vice-President of the International Association for Forensic Psychotherapy.

Gwen Adshead is a forensic psychiatrist and psychotherapist. She trained at St George's Hospital, the Institute of Psychiatry and the Institute of Group Analysis. She also has a research interest in attachment theory applied to forensic psychiatric services. She has been a consultant forensic psychotherapist at Broadmoor Hospital for over ten years, where she runs therapy groups for offenders. She is also a regular teacher, lecturer and writer: she has written over 100 papers and book chapters on a variety of topics including forensic psychotherapy, attachment theory and ethics in mental health. She is currently training as a mindfulness teacher, and working on a book about evil. She is also currently President of the International Association for Forensic Psychotherapy.

Anne Aiyegbusi is Deputy Director of Nursing, Specialist and Forensic Services, West London Mental Health NHS Trust. She has worked for many years in forensic mental health nursing in a range of registered nursing roles and grades, including that of consultant nurse for women's secure services. She has worked across the range of secure mental health settings, including two high secure hospitals. Her main clinical interest is in integrating attachment theory principles into forensic mental health nursing. She is also interested in the manifestation of early traumatic experience in the lives of service users, and in particular, how this reverberates throughout the care system. She has published widely and made many conference presentations about the psychodynamics of forensic mental health nursing. She completed her PhD in 2011 and her thesis focused on the therapeutic relationship between nurse and service users diagnosed with personality disorders. She is currently Secretary of the International Association for Forensic Psychotherapy.

Tom Clarke is Associate Director of Nursing with South West London and St George's Mental Health NHS Trust and honorary lecturer at Kingston University. He is the developer and CEO of POEThealth Ltd, an integrated approach to the functional design evaluation of inpatient environments.

Jonathan Coe is Managing Director of the Clinic for Boundaries Studies. Previously he was CEO of the charity WITNESS (POPAN). He recently completed a Winston Churchill Trust travelling fellowship study tour to the USA where he visited a wide range of organisations involved in work around professional boundary violations. He acted as a lay member of the Expert Advisory Group for the National Operating Standards for psychological therapies, the Department of Health working group on the Statutory Regulation of Herbal Medicine, Acupuncture and Traditional Chinese Medicine and the Ethics Committee of the British Psychological Society. He was a member of the steering group for the CHRE Clear Sexual Boundaries project and was a lay member of the Health Professions Council Professional Liaison Group on the regulation of counsellors and psychotherapists. He has worked in mental health services for the last 24 years.

Andrew Cooper is Professor of Social Work at the Tavistock Clinic and University of East London, and a psychoanalytic psychotherapist in private practice. He has written widely about contemporary child protection, the societal role of social work and some of the sources of its afflictions. He runs the Tavistock/UEL Professional Doctorate in Social Work and co-ordinates the Tavistock Policy Seminar series.

With Julian Lousada he wrote *Borderline Welfare: Feeling and Fear of Feeling in Modern Welfare* (Karnac Books 2005).

Alan Corbett is a Psychoanalytic Psychotherapist with training in Psychotherapy (Guild of Psychotherapists, London), Forensic Psychotherapy (Tavistock and Portman Trust, London), Clinical Supervision (Guild of Psychotherapists, London) and Child Psychotherapy (Children's Therapy Centre, Ireland). He was Director of Respond, UK, a clinic for people with intellectual disabilities who have experienced and/or perpetrated sexual abuse, before becoming National Clinical Director of the CARI (Children at Risk in Ireland) Foundation. He is a Member of the Guild of Psychotherapists, the British Association of Psychoanalytic and Psychodynamic Supervision, the Institute of Psychotherapy and Disability and is registered with the UKCP. He is a Member of the Board of the International Association for Forensic Psychotherapy, a Trustee of the Institute of Psychotherapy and Disability and a Council Member of the Guild of Psychotherapists. In addition to providing psychotherapy for children and adults with and without disabilities, he provides forensic assessments for court, and lectures on psychotherapy, disability and sexual trauma and is a lecturer on the An Garda Síochána Specialist Child Interviewing training course and on the MSc in Psychoanalytic Psychotherapy at Trinity College Dublin. He is currently undertaking doctoral research into consent issues relating to people with intellectual disability (University of Kent).

Earl Hopper is a psychoanalyst, group analyst and organisational consultant in private practice in London. He is a Fellow of the British Psychoanalytical Society, a member of the Institute of Group Analysis, a full member of the Group Analytic Society (London), and a Fellow of the American Group Psychotherapy Association. He is a supervisor and training analyst for the Institute of Group Analysis, the British Association of Psychotherapists and the London Centre for Psychotherapy. He is also an Honorary Tutor at The Tavistock and Portman NHS Trust and a member of the Faculty of the Post-Doctoral Program at Adelphi University, New York. He is a former President of the International Association for Group Psychotherapy and Group Processes (IAGP) and a former Chairman of the Association of Independent Psychoanalysts of the British Psychoanalytical Society. He is the Editor of the New International Library of Group Analysis.

Pam Kleinot is a psychoanalytic psychotherapist and group analyst at City and Hackney Psychotherapy Department. She runs groups at Newham Psychological Services and works at the Discovery Project in Tower Hamlets, a day therapeutic community for people suffering long-term psychotic illness. She formerly worked at HMP Holloway and the Women's Therapy Centre. She is a former sub-editor on the *Guardian* newspaper and is executive editor of the journal *Group Analysis*. She is a member of the Arbours Association, the Institute of Group Analysis and was formerly a Board member of the International Association for Forensic Psychotherapy.

Anna Motz is Consultant Clinical and Forensic Psychologist at Thames Valley Forensic Mental Health Services and Psychotherapist in training at the Tavistock Clinic. She is the author of *The Psychology of Female Violence, Crimes Against the Body* (Routledge 2001, Second Edition 2008), editor of *Managing Self Harm: Psychological Perspectives* (Routledge 2009) and author of the forthcoming book *Toxic Couples: The Psychology of Violent Relationships* (Routledge 2012). She has extensive experience of the assessment and treatment of perpetrators and victims of violence and of consulting to the staff teams who work with them.

Rebecca Neeld is a group psychotherapist at the Cassel Hospital, West London Mental Health NHS Trust. She has a special interest in services for people with personality disorders.

Kingsley Norton qualified in medicine at Clare College, Cambridge, thereafter pursuing a career in psychiatry at St George's, London, and obtaining his MD (Cantab) in 1988. He qualified as a Jungian Analyst in 1989 (Society of Analytical Psychologists) and has held Consultant appointments in General Psychiatry (1984–89) and in Psychotherapy (Henderson Hospital, 1986–2006, as Director; and West London Mental Health Trust, 2006 to date). He has written and researched extensively in the fields of Personality Disorder, Therapeutic Communities, and healthcare organisation. He has written/co-written four books. The last, *Setting up Services in the NHS* (Jessica Kingsley Publishers 2006), describes the processes involved in leading the successful project to propagate the Henderson Hospital Therapeutic Community method of treatment for personality disordered patients to the Midlands and North-West of England. As clinical lead for personality disorder in his current post, he remains committed to improving the service received by people diagnosed with personality disorder, leading the development of a Trust-wide managed clinical network for these service users.

Stanley Ruszczynski is a Consultant Adult Psychotherapist and Clinical Director of the Portman Clinic (Tavistock and Portman NHS Foundation Trust), London, an NHS forensic psychotherapy clinic. He is a psychoanalyst and individual and couple psychoanalytic psychotherapist, and is a full member of the British Psychoanalytic Association, the British Association of Psychotherapists and the British Society of Couple Psychotherapists and Counsellors. He was previously Deputy Director and both Clinical and Training Co-ordinator at the Tavistock Centre for Couple Relationships. He teaches, lectures and undertakes organisational consultancy in the UK and abroad and is the author of 30 book chapters and journal articles and has edited and co-edited five books, the most recent being *Lectures on Violence, Perversion and Delinquency* (Karnac Books 2007), co-edited with David Morgan.

Christopher Scanlon is Consultant Psychotherapist in general adult and forensic mental health with the lead for group psychotherapy, and for reflective practice and team development, Department of Psychotherapy, St Thomas' Hospital, London; Training Group Analyst and member of Faculty Institute of Group Analysis (London); Senior Visiting Research Fellow at the Centre for Psycho-social Studies, University of West England (UWE); an associate of the Organisation for the Promotion of the Understanding of Society (OPUS); and member of the International Society for the Psychoanalytic Study of Organizations (ISPSO). He was previously Consultant Psychotherapist and lead for Training and Consultation at Henderson Hospital Democratic Therapeutic Community Services, professional adviser to the Department of Health's Personality Disorder Expert Advisory Group and a trustee of the Zito Trust – a major UK Mental Health Charity campaigning for improved services for mentally disordered offenders and their victims.

Valerie Sinason is a poet, writer, child and adult psychotherapist and psychoanalyst. She is President of the Institute for Psychotherapy and Disability and Director of the Clinic for Dissociative Studies. Her latest book *Trauma, Dissociation and Multiplicity, Working with Identity and Selves* has just been published by Routledge (2011).

Celia Taylor trained in Forensic Psychiatry at the Institute of Psychiatry in London. Between 1995 and 1997 she was an Honorary Senior Lecturer at the Institute of Psychiatry and Consultant Forensic Psychiatrist at Broadmoor Hospital. She then worked in the private sector for five years, setting up a medium secure personality disorder unit. During this time she was involved in an evaluation of Close Supervision Centres (special units for the most violent prison inmates), funded and published by the Home Office. In November 2003 she returned to the NHS to set up one of three national pilot medium secure 'Dangerous and Severe Personality Disorder' services initiated by the Ministry of Justice and Department of Health. The Millfields Unit is based on the campus of the John Howard Centre in Hackney and has 20 beds for adult men and 75 staff. The treatment model is that of a modified therapeutic community. She is overseeing research into the characteristics of the first 200 referrals as well as a systematic review of the impact of this work upon staff. She is also regularly involved in conducting peer reviews of papers submitted to journals in the field. She is currently Vice-President of the International Association for Forensic Psychotherapy.

Estela Welldon is the Founder and Honorary Elected President for Life of the International Association for Forensic Psychotherapy, a Fellow of the Royal College of Psychiatrists, an Honorary Consultant Psychiatrist in Psychotherapy at the Tavistock Clinic and the Portman Clinic, a Senior Member of the British Association for Psychotherapy, the American Group Psychotherapy Association, the International Association of Group Psychotherapy and of the Confederation of British Psychotherapists. She is an honorary member of the Institute of Group Analysis and of the Society of Couple Psychoanalytic Psychotherapists, Tavistock Clinic. In 1997 she was awarded an Honorary Doctorate of Science degree by Oxford Brookes University for her contributions to the field of forensic psychotherapy. She is the author of *Mother, Madonna, Whore: the*

Idealization and Denigration of Motherhood (1988) which has been translated into many languages; *Sadomasochism* (2002); *Playing with Dynamite: A personal approach to the psychoanalytic understanding of Perversion, Violence and Criminality* (2011); and is co-editor of *A Practical Guide to Forensic Psychotherapy* (1997). She works privately as a psychoanalytic psychotherapist. She is a sought-after lecturer worldwide. Her subjects include male and female perversions, forensic psychotherapy and group analytic psychotherapy.

Martin Wrench is Associate Director of Social Work in the Specialist Services Directorate at South West London and St George's NHS Mental Health Trust. He was Principal Social Worker in a Forensic Service between 1989 and 1999 and Principal Social Worker at the Henderson Hospital, a residential democratic therapeutic community for people with personality disorder, from 1999 until 2010. Martin is an experienced trainer in mental health and has developed and taught on a range of courses relating to personality disorder for professionals working in the voluntary sector, criminal justice, social care and the NHS. He has over 20 years' experience of consulting to organisations, teams and individual practitioners and clinicians and has written articles on a range of topics which include consultation to staff providing sex offender treatment, mental health law and the role of the forensic social worker. Martin is also a cognitive analytic psychotherapist.

SUBJECT INDEX

AUTHOR INDEX